Last Minute Resources for MRCOG 1 Exam

A Compilation of One-Liners, Tables for Last Minute Glance and Mnemonics

Last Minute Resources for MRCOG 1 Exam

A Compilation of One-Liners, Tables for Last Minute Glance and Mnemonics

Richa Saxena
Obsteetrician Gynaecologist
MBBS MD (Obstetrics and Gynecology)
PG Diploma in Clinical Research
New Delhi, India

Copyright © 2018 Richa Saxena.
ISBN: (Softcover) 978-1986709781

All rights reserved. No part of this book may be used or reproduced by any means, graphic, electronic, or mechanical, including photocopying, recording, taping or by any information storage retrieval system without the written permission of the author except in the case of brief quotations embodied in critical articles and reviews.
Because of the dynamic nature of the internet, any web addresses or links contained in this book may have changed since publication and may no longer be valid. The views expressed in this work are solely those of the author and do not necessarily reflect the views of the publisher, and the publisher hereby disclaims any responsibility for them.
Cover photo Courtesy: Mongyu Marma
To contact the author, kindly visit her website www.drrichasaxena.com.
Alternatively, you can email her at richa@drrichasaxena.com.

PREFACE

While preparing for the MRCOG part 1 exam, each student on an average requires 3 to 6 months of time to build up their concepts, get familiar with the exam pattern and practice SBAs (single best answers). However, just a week prior to the exam they need to focus on remembering and memorising all these important concepts and details. This book is likely to help the students in just achieving this. It is not a comprehensive textbook, rather a concise ready reckoner for a quick glance just before the exam.

It would act as a guide for last minute revision prior to the MRCOG, part 1 exam. The book comprises of more than 1,000 one-liners in all, including subjects such as anatomy, physiology, biochemistry, embryology, pathology, microbiology, genetics, pharmacology, endocrinology, biophysics, biostatistics, obstetrics and gynaecology. The one-liners are likely to be useful for the students because they are based on the SBAs asked in the MRCOG exam over the past 5 years and are built on the concept that the student is required to choose the best answer for a question having the SBA format. If he or she already know the best answer, they are likely to choose the correct answer amongst the given options.

There is another section comprising of tables for quick glances. This contains information, which has been designed in form of a table. This would help in quick revision just prior to the exam.

Use of mnemonics is another educational aid, which is likely to strengthen a candidate's memory, thereby assisting them to memorize important facts before the examination. Similar to the one-liners and quick glances, mnemonics too have been categorized subject-wise, thereby covering the entire syllabus.

Writing a book is a colossal task. It cannot be completed without divine intervention and approval. Therefore, I have decided to end this preface with a small prayer of thanks to the Almighty which I was taught in the childhood.

*"Father lead me day by day, ever in thy own sweet way.
Teach me to be pure and good and tell me what I ought to do"*
–Amen

Simultaneously, I would like to extend my thanks and appreciation to all the related authors and publishers whose references have been used in this book. Though extreme care has been taken to maintain the accuracy while writing this book, constructive criticism would be greatly appreciated. Please email me your comments at richa@drrichasaxena.com. Also, please feel free to visit my website www.drrichasaxena.com for obtaining information related to various books written by me and to make use of the free resources available for the MRCOG candidates.

Richa Saxena
richa@drrichasaxena.com
www.drrichasaxena.com

Contents

Section 1: One-Liner Questions
1. Anatomy...9
2. Physiology..31
3. Biochemistry..57
4. Pathology...71
5. Microbiology...81
6. Immunology..97
7. Embryology...115
8. Genetics...127
9. Biophysics...141
10. Epidemiology and Biostatistics......................151
11. Pharmacology..171
12. Obstetrics...195
13. Gynaecology 221
14. Endocrinology...245

Section 2: Last minute glance
15. Anatomy..265
16. Physiology...277
17. Biochemistry...283
18. Pathology...289
19. Microbiology...299
20. Immunology..307
21. Embryology 311
22. Genetics...315
23. Biophysics 319
24. Epidemiology..321
25. Pharmacology..323
26. Obstetrics...333
27. Gynaecology..343
28. Endocrinology...351

Section 3: Appendix
29. Mnemonics..359

LAST MINUTE RESOURCES FOR MRCOG 1

ONE-LINER QUESTIONS
CHAPTER 1
Anatomy

Q: At which level the abdominal aorta divides into two common iliac?
Ans: The abdominal aorta ends by dividing into two common iliac arteries at the level of L4.

Q: Which ascending artery can be damaged during open appendectomy?
Ans: Deep circumflex artery

Q: When you hold the bony pelvis in anatomical position which two landmarks are at the same level horizontally?
Ans: Symphysis pubis and ischial spine

Q: What is the submento-bregmatic diameter?
Ans: 9.4 cm

Q: What makes a dimple in the gluteal region?
Ans: Posterior superior iliac spine

Q: What is the type of cells lining labia majora?
Ans: Keratinized stratified squamous

Q: Anterior fontanelle closes at what age?
Ans: Approximately 18months

Q: What is the timing for chorionic villus sampling (CVS)?
Ans: 10–12 weeks of gestation

Q: What is the timing for amniocentesis?
Ans: 16–20 weeks of gestation

Q: Which nerve pass through rectus sheath?
Ans: Subcostal nerve

Q: Which lymph node is involved in most of the cases of testicular cancer?
Ans: Para-aortic lymph node

Q: What is the level of bifurcation of aorta?
Ans: Uppermost edge of iliac crest

Q: What is the narrowest portion of fallopian tube?
Ans: Isthmus

Q: What is the nerve root of ilioinguinal and iliohypogastric nerve?
Ans: L1

Q: What is blood supply of Bartholin's gland?
Ans: Deep external pudendal artery

Q: Which muscles are cut during a mediolateral episiotomy?
Ans: Bulbospongiosus and superficial transverse perineal muscles

Q: Which layer of adrenal cortex release glucocorticoids?
Ans: Zona fasciculate

Q: What is the nerve supply to the skin of the perineum?
Ans: Inferior rectal

Q: Which structure demarcates external iliac artery and femoral artery?
Ans: Inguinal ligament

Q: The round ligament of the uterus develops from which embryonic structure?
Ans: Gubernaculum

Q: Which structure is the principle supports of the uterus?
Ans: Transverse cervical ligament

Q: Which structure separates the superficial perineal pouch from the deep perineal pouch?
Ans: Perineal membrane

ONE-LINER QUESTIONS

Q: Which screening test has high negative predictive value for detection of pre-term pre-labour rupture of the membranes?
Ans: Foetal fibronectin test

Q: Which structure blocks the blood supply to a loop of small intestine at the femoral ring causing strangulated femoral hernia?
Ans: Lacunar ligament

Q: What is the anatomical location of Bartholin's gland?
Ans: Superficial perineal pouch

Q: Sympathetic supply to the urinary bladder is derived from which lumbar segments?
Ans: L1 and L2

Q: What is the approximate expected angle between the brim of the pelvis to the horizontal plane, when the body is in the upright position.
Ans: 60 degrees

Q: What is the relationship between pudendal nerve and pudendal artery?
Ans: Pudendal nerve is medial to pudendal artery

Q: Which structure develops into kidney and renal duct?
Ans: Metanephros

Q: At which level the abdominal aorta divides into two common iliac?
Ans. The abdominal aorta ends by dividing into two common iliac arteries at the level of L4.

Q: When you hold the bony pelvis in anatomical position which two landmarks are at the same level horizontally?
Ans: Symphysis pubis and ischial spine

Q: What makes a dimple in the gluteal region?

Ans: Posterior superior iliac spine

Q: What is the type of cells lining labia majora?
Ans: Keratinized stratified squamous

Q: Which is the most common anatomical location for appendix?
Ans: Retrocaecal

Q: Appendix receives its blood supply from which branch of the posterior caecal artery?
Ans: Appendicular artery

Q: Which structure crosses the right ureter in the pelvis and where?
Ans: Crossed by common iliac vessels at sacroiliac joint

Q: What kind of joint is the hip joint?
Ans: Synovial joint

Q: What kind of joint is the pubic symphysis?
Ans: Cartilaginous joint

Q: Which structure enters inguinal canal and is identified easily at laparoscopy?
Ans: Round ligament

Q: Which nerve supplies posterior two-third of labia majora?
Ans: Perineal nerve (branch of pudendal)

Q: Which artery supplies blood to rectus abdominis muscle below umbilicus?
Ans: Inferior epigastric artery

Q: Which structure is attached to anterior superior iliac spine?
Ans: Inguinal ligament

Q: If the mandible is undeveloped, which structure is likely to be damaged?
Ans: Facial nerve

ONE-LINER QUESTIONS

Q: What is the nerve root of ilioinguinal and iliohypogastric nerve?
Ans: L1

Q: Which type of epithelium lines the lower urethra near the external urethral orifice?
Ans: Stratified squamous non-keratinized type

Q: At what vertebral level is the umbilicus?
Ans: L3-L4

Q: The ureter crosses in front of the internal iliac artery at what level?
Ans: Sacroiliac joint

Q: Which structure is the principle support of the uterus?
Ans: Transverse cervical ligament

Q: The posterior fontanelle usually closes by what age?
Ans: 3 months

Q: Which nerve or nerve plexus provides sensory innervation to the cervix?
Ans: Pelvic splanchnic nerve

Q: The greater omentum is derived from which embryonic structure?
Ans: Dorsal mesogastrium

Q: From which posterior division structure of endoderm does the rectum originates?
Ans: Primitive cloaca

Q: What kind of embryological defect results in imperforate anus?
Ans: Imperforate anus occurs due to the failure of the cloacal membrane to break down.

Q: At the level of which structure does the bifurcation of the abdominal aorta occur?
Ans: Highest point of iliac crest

Q: What is the correct order of musculature of the anal canal from deep to superficial?
Ans: The correct order of musculature of the anal canal from deep to superficial is as follows:
1. Internal sphincter
2. Deep part of external sphincter
3. Superficial part of external sphincter
4. Subcutaneous part of external sphincter

Q: Which vessels can possibly be injured in the subcutaneous tissue when a transverse suprapubic skin incision is made?
Ans: Superficial epigastric vessels.

Q: What is the embryological origin of the round ligament of the uterus?
Ans. Gubernaculum ovarii

Q: Where does the round ligament of the uterus originate from?
Ans: Anteroinferior to uterine cornua

Q: What is the ending of the round ligament of the uterus?
Ans: Labium majus

Q: Which of nerve pierces the internal oblique muscle and passes through the inguinal canal?
Ans: Ilioinguinal nerve

Q: Which nerve is likely to be affected after an ovarian surgery patient felt pain at the right side of thigh?
Ans: Obturator nerve

Q: Name the structure that leaves through lesser sciatic foramen?
Ans: Tendon of obturator internus

Q: Which nerve passes over psoas major muscle?
Ans: Genitofemoral nerve
Q: Ovarian artery is a branch of which aorta?

ONE-LINER QUESTIONS

Ans: Abdominal aorta

Q: The abdominal aorta bifurcates into two common iliac arteries at the level of which lumbar vertebra?
Ans: L4

Q: At which level the ovarian artery arises from the abdominal aorta?
Ans: L2

Q: Which artery supplies the anorectal canal superior to the pectinate line?
Ans: Inferior mesenteric artery

Q: Which is the arterial supply of the anorectal canal inferior to the pectinate line?
Ans: Internal pudendal artery

Q: What is the anatomical location of Bartholin's gland?
Ans: Superficial perineal pouch

Q: Sympathetic supply to the urinary bladder is derived from which lumbar segments?
Ans. L1 and L2

Q: Which part of the female urogenital system describes the vestibule?
Ans: Space between labium minora

Q: Which artery supplies the structures derived from the midgut of the embryo?
Ans. Superior mesenteric artery

Q: Motor fibres to detrusor muscle of the urinary bladder are derived from which nerve?
Ans: Pelvic splanchnic nerve plexus

Q: Which of the following muscles leaves the lesser pelvis through the greater sciatic foramen?
Ans: Piriformis

Q: Which of the following nerves enters the thigh by passing beneath the inguinal ligament, just medial to the anterior superior iliac spine?
Ans: Lateral cutaneous nerve of thigh

Q: What landmark marks the point where the external iliac artery becomes the femoral artery?
Ans: Inguinal ligament

Q: What is the blood supply of sigmoid colon?
Ans: Inferior mesenteric artery

Q: Which structure forms the lateral wall of the ischiorectal fossa?
Ans: Obturator internus fascia

Q: At what level does ovarian artery arise?
Ans: L2

Q: What is the relation of femoral nerve with femoral artery and vein from lateral to medial?
Ans: Nerve-Artery-Vein

Q: Of which artery are the arteries, dorsal artery of clitoris and deep artery of clitoris branches of?
Ans: Internal pudendal artery

Q: What is the dermatome level at suprapubic incision?
Ans: L1

Q: What is the level of dermatome for epidural at umbilical region?
Ans: T10/

Q: What is the level of dermatome for nipples?
Ans: T4

ONE-LINER QUESTIONS

Q: What is the nerve supply of external anal sphincter?
Ans: Pudendal nerve

Q: Which structure in female is homologous to male prostate?
Ans: Skene's gland

Q: What is pudendal cleft?
Ans: The pudendal cleft is a part of the vulva, the furrow at the base of the mons pubis where it divides to form the labia majora.

Q: Which nerve supplies pyramidalis?
Ans: Subcostal nerve

Q: Which artery can be damaged during sacrospinous ligament fixation?
Ans: Internal pudendal artery

Q: Which is the direct branch of superior vesicle artery?
Ans: Anterior division of internal iliac artery

Q: The medial umbilical ligament is a remnant of what structure?
Ans: Urachus

Q: What is the origin of anterior cerebral artery?
Ans: The internal carotid artery

Q: What is the origin of middle cerebral artery?
Ans: Anterior cerebral artery

Q: What is the origin of vertebral arteries?
Ans: Subclavian artery branches in to vertebral arteries.

Q: What is the origin of basilar artery?
Ans: Vertebral arteries fuse to form basilar artery.

Q: Where is aortic aperture located?
Ans: Behind median arcuate ligament and in front of disc between vertebrae T12 and L1.

Q: What structures pass through aortic aperture?
Ans: Aorta, thoracic duct, azygos and hemiazygos veins.

Q: Where is aperture for the oesophagus located?
Ans: At the level of 10th thoracic vertebra.

Q: What passes through aperture for the oesophagus?
Ans: Oesophagus; phrenooesophageal ligament; the vagal trunks; the right and left gastric nerves; and oesophageal branches of the left gastric artery, with their accompanying veins and lymphatics.

Q: Where is aperture for the inferior vena cava?
Ans: The inferior vena cava enters through the opening opposite the T8 vertebra.

Q: What is motor supply of diaphragm?
Ans: The right and left phrenic nerves.

Q: What is sensory supply of diaphragm?
Ans: From lower six intercostal nerves.

Q: What are the main types of arteries that *supply* blood to the *diaphragm*?
Ans: Right and left phrenic arteries; the intercostal arteries; and the musculophrenic branches of the internal thoracic arteries.

Q: Mention the venous supply of diaphragm.
Ans: Inferior vena cava and azygos vein (on the right) and the adrenal/renal and hemiazygos veins (on the left).

Q: From which nerve roots does phrenic nerve arises?
Ans: Each phrenic nerve arises from the spinal nerves C3, C4 and C5. Contribution from C4 is the greatest.

Q: Name the most common site of breast carcinomas.
Ans: Upper outer quadrant of the breast (containing a large amount of glandular tissue).

Q: Mention arterial supply to the breast.

ONE-LINER QUESTIONS

Ans: Axillary artery (via branches like superior thoracic artery, pectoral branches of thoracoacromial artery, lateral thoracic artery, etc.); internal thoracic artery; and intercostal arteries.

Q: Mention lymphatic drainage of superolateral quadrant of breast.
Ans: Anterior, posterior axillary group of lymph nodes and supraclavicular group of lymph nodes.

Q: Mention lymphatic drainage of superomedial quadrant.
Ans: Internal mammary group, supraclavicular nodes.

Q: Mention lymphatic drainage of inferomedial quadrant.
Ans: Internal mammary group, supradiaphragmatic nodes.

Q: Mention lymphatic drainage of inferolateral quadrant.
Ans: Posterior intercostal nodes, subdiaphragmatic group.

Q: Which nerves supply the breast?
Ans: 4th–6th intercostal nerves.

Q: What is the direction of fibres of external oblique muscles?
Ans: Fibres of the external oblique muscle run forwards and downwards.

Q: What is the direction of fibres of internal oblique muscles?
Ans: The fibres of the internal oblique muscle run forwards and upwards.

Q: Which abdominal muscle produces a six-pack appearance?
Ans: Rectus Abdominis muscle

Q: What is the origin of Superior epigastric vessel?
Ans: It is direct continuation of the internal thoracic artery.

Q: What is the origin of inferior epigastric vessel?
Ans: It arises from the external iliac artery just superior to the inguinal ligaments.

Q: What is the origin of superficial circumflex iliac artery?
Ans: It is the branch of femoral artery.

Q: What is the nerve supply to the skin superior to the umbilicus?
Ans: Supplied by T7–T9.

Q: What is the nerve supply to the skin around the umbilicus?
Ans: Supplied by T10.

Q: What is the nerve supply to the skin below the umbilicus?
Ans: Supplied by T11 and the cutaneous branches of the subcostal, iliohypogastric and ilioinguinal nerves.

Q: What is composition of anterior/upper layer of rectus sheath above the arcuate line?
Ans: Anterior lamina of internal oblique aponeurosis and aponeurosis of external oblique

Q: What is composition of anterior/upper layer of rectus sheath below the arcuate line?
Ans: Aponeurosis of three flat muscles of abdomen:
1. External oblique
2. Internal oblique
3. Transversus abdominis

Q: What is composition of posterior/lower layer of rectus sheath above the arcuate line?
Ans: The posterior/lower layer of rectus sheath above the arcuate line is composed of the following structures:
1. Posterior lamina of the internal oblique muscle
2. Aponeurosis of transversus abdominis

Q: What is composition of posterior/lower layer of rectus sheath below the arcuate line?
Ans: Transversalis fascia

Q: What forms anterior boundary of Epiploic foramen?
Ans: Free border of the lesser omentum, along with the common bile duct, hepatic artery, and portal vein between its two layers.

ONE-LINER QUESTIONS

Q: What forms posterior boundary of Epiploic foramen?
Ans: Peritoneum covering the inferior vena cava.

Q: What forms superior boundary of Epiploic foramen?
Ans: The peritoneum on the caudate lobe of the liver.

Q: What forms inferior boundary of Epiploic foramen?
Ans: Peritoneum, which covers the first part of the duodenum and the hepatic artery. The hepatic artery passes forward below the foramen before ascending between the two layers of the lesser omentum.

Q: What forms the superior wall (roof) of inguinal canal?
Ans: Medial crus of aponeurosis of external oblique; musculoaponeurotic arches of internal oblique and transversus abdominis; and transversalis fascia.

Q: What forms the anterior wall of inguinal canal?
Ans: Aponeurosis of the external oblique (in the medial third), and fleshy part of internal oblique (lateral third of canal only).

Q: What forms the posterior wall of inguinal canal?
Ans: The posterior wall of inguinal ligament is composed of the following structures:
1. Transversalis fascia
2. Medial-third of the posterior wall: Conjoint tendon (fused aponeuroses of the internal oblique and transversus abdominis), and inguinal falx (reflected part of inguinal ligament)
3. Lateral-third of the posterior wall: Deep inguinal ring

Q: What forms the inferior wall (floor) of inguinal canal?
Ans: Inguinal ligament; lacunar ligament (medial-third of canal only); and iliopubic tract (lateral-third of canal only).

Q: In males, what are the contents of the inguinal canal?
Ans: Spermatic cord and ilioinguinal nerve (this nerve only passes through the superficial inguinal ring). This nerve is not carried through the deep inguinal ring and therefore does not formally

travel through the inguinal canal).

Q: In females, what are the contents of the inguinal canal?
Ans: Round ligament (in the female the inguinal canal transmits the round ligament to the labium majus) and ilioinguinal nerve (this nerve only passes through the superficial inguinal ring. It is not carried through the deep inguinal ring).

Q: What is the location of inguinal ligament?
Ans: At the upper end of the front of the thigh, i.e. at its junction with the anterior abdominal wall

Q: What is the composition of inguinal ligament?
Ans: It is the thickened and folded lower edge of the aponeurosis of the external oblique muscle.

Q: What is the origin and end of inguinal ligament?
Ans: It extends from the anterior superior iliac spine to the pubic tubercle.

Q: What is spermatic cord?
Ans: It is formed when testis passes through the inguinal canal descending into the scrotum.
Q: Name the three coverings of spermatic cord.
Ans: Internal spermatic fascia; cremasteric fascia; and external spermatic fascia.

Q: What are contents of spermatic cord?
Ans: Vas deferens (ductus deferens); three nerves (genital branch of genitofemoral nerve, ilioinguinal nerve, and sympathetic nerves); three arteries (testicular artery, artery to the vas, and cremasteric artery); lymphatics (which drain to the para-aortic nodes); pampiniform venous plexus; and processus vaginalis.

Q: Which nerve roots emerge from the pelvic sacral foramina?
Ans: Ventral rami of S1–S4.

Q: What is the extent of sacrospinous ligament?
Ans: Extends from the lateral margin of the sacrum and coccyx to

the ischial spine.

Q: What is the extent of sacrotuberous ligament?
Ans: Extends from the sacrum to the ischial tuberosity.

Q: How is the shape of sacrum in a gynaecoid pelvis in females opposed from that in the male pelvis?
Ans: Sacrum in a gynaecoid pelvis is broad, shallow, and concave, as opposed to the flattened, narrow, and long sacrum in the male pelvis.

Q: What is the nerve supply to the external genitalia?
Ans: The nerves which supply the external genitalia include the following:
1. Pudendal nerve (which arises at S2-S4 levels and accompanies the pudendal vessels)
2. Ilioinguinal (L1) and the genital branch of the genitofemoral (L1-L2), arising from the lumbar plexus, innervate the medial and lateral aspects of the vulvar skin, respectively.

Q: What kind of epithelium lines the vaginal mucosa?
Ans: Stratified squamous epithelium

Q: What is arterial supply of vagina?
Ans: Uterine and vaginal branches of the internal iliac artery and inferior vesical and middle rectal arteries.

Q: What is venous supply of vagina?
Ans: Venous drainage of vagina is to the vaginal venous plexus with the vaginal vein draining into the internal iliac vein or the uterine vein.

Q: Mention lymphatic drainage of the lower one-third of the vagina.
Ans: Drains to the superficial inguinal lymph nodes.

Q: Mention lymphatic drainage of the upper one-third of the vagina.
Ans: Drain into the external and internal iliac and sacral nodes

Q: Describe peritoneal relations of Fallopian tube.
Ans: The Fallopian tube runs in the upper margin of the broad ligament (part of which is known as the mesosalpinx). It encloses the tube in such a way that it is completely covered with peritoneum except for a narrow strip along its inferior aspect.

Q: What is the widest and the largest part of the Fallopian tube?
Ans: Ampulla

Q: Where does fertilization of oocyte normally occurs inside the Fallopian tube?
Ans: Ampulla

Q: What structures are related to the ovarian fossa?
Ans: The relationships of ovarian fossa are as follows:
Superiorly: External iliac vessels
Anteriorly: Obliterated umbilical artery
Posteriorly: Ureter and internal iliac artery.

Q: Define relationship between the size of uterine body and cervix in an adult and a newborn.
Ans: In an adult woman, the uterine body is twice as long as the cervix, while the opposite is true in the newborn.

Q: Where does the round ligament ends?
Ans: Labium majus

Q: Define relationship between the size of uterine corpus and cervix during reproductive years.
Ans: The corpus is twice as long as the cervix.

Q: Define relationship between the size of uterine corpus and cervix after menopause.
Ans: The cervix is twice as long as the uterine corpus.

Q: What is length of cervix in an adult non-pregnant woman?
Ans: 2.5 cm

Q: At what level does the external os of cervix lie?

ONE-LINER QUESTIONS

Ans: On a level with the ischial spines.

Q: What kind of epithelium lines the ectocervix?
Ans: Stratified squamous epithelium

Q: What kind of epithelium lines the endocervix?
Ans: Simple columnar epithelium

Q: What is the location of squamo-columnar junction after the menopause?
Ans: It usually recedes within the endocervical canal.

Q: What is the location of squamo-columnar junction at puberty?
Ans: It extends distally into the vagina.

Q: Which is the most common site of cervical carcinoma?
Ans: Transformation zone

Q: What is the consistency of cervical mucus during various phases of menstrual cycle?
Ans: *Before ovulation*: Consistency of mucus is thick and impenetrable to sperms.
At ovulation: Consistency changes as it becomes more thin and stretchable (sperms can penetrate through it and fertilisation can occur).

Q: Mention the peritoneal relations of supravaginal portion of cervix.
Ans: *Anteriorly*: Not covered by the peritoneum
Posteriorly: Peritoneum covers supravaginal cervix and the upper-third of the posterior vaginal wall.

Q: What is the blood supply to the uterus?
Ans: Uterine artery (one on each side). It is a branch of the anterior trunk of the internal iliac artery.

Q: What is the relation between uterine artery and ureter?
Ans: Uterine artery crosses above the ureter at a distance of about 2 cm from the uterus, at the level of the internal os. The ureter,

therefore, passes under the uterine artery.

Q: During second trimester in normal pregnancy, which vessels are responsible for a 10-fold increase in blood flow?
Ans: Spiral vessels

Q: What is the action of alpha-receptors and beta-receptors on uterine musculature?
Ans: *Alpha-receptors*: Cause contractions in the pregnant uterus
Beta-receptors: Cause relaxation in the non-pregnant uterus.

Q: Define lymphatic drainage of the fundus and upper part of the uterine body.
Ans: Drain into the lumbar (aortic) nodes.

Q: Define lymphatic drainage of lowest part of the uterine body.
Ans: Drain into the external iliac nodes.

Q: Define lymphatic drainage of cervix.
Ans: Drains into the external and internal iliac and the sacral nodes.

Q: Define alternative lymphatic drainage of uterine fundus.
Ans: Few vessels at the fundus follow the ovarian channels, and there is an inconstant pathway along the round ligament to the superficial inguinal group of lymph nodes.

Q: What are the functions of testis?
Ans: Producing sperms and male hormones (mainly testosterone), which regulate reproductive organ development.

Q: How long spermatogenesis takes?
Ans: 74 ± 4 Days.

Q: What is the main site of testosterone synthesis?
Ans: Leydig cell of testis

Q: Which hormone stimulates the production of testosterone?
Ans: Luteinising hormone

ONE-LINER QUESTIONS

Q: What is action of inhibin?
Ans: It down regulates FSH synthesis and inhibits its secretion.

Q: Where is inhibin synthesised?
Ans: Sertoli cell

Q: Define lymphatic drainage of testis.
Ans: Drains to the para-aortic group of lymph nodes in the region of the renal arteries.

Q: How is structure of the rectum is different from that of the colon?
Ans: Absence of taenia coli; sacculations; and appendices epiploicae.

Q: Which vertebra corresponds to the termination of a definite mesentery?
Ans: The third sacral vertebra

Q: Mention the peritoneal relations of rectum.
Ans: *Upper part of the rectum*: Covered with peritoneum in front and at the sides
Middle part: Covered in front only
Lower part: Devoid of peritoneal covering.

Q: What is blood supply of rectum?
Ans: Inferior mesenteric artery through its rectal branches.

Q: What is nerve supply of rectum?
Ans: Its parasympathetic supply is derived from the hypogastric plexus of S234 origin.

Q: What is lymphatic drainage of rectum?
Ans: Drains into the internal and common iliac nodes; the sacral nodes; and along the superior arteries in to the pre-aortic nodes.

Q: What is length of anal canal?
Ans: 4 cm

Q: What is the direction of lower part of the rectum?
Ans: Directed downwards and forwards.

Q: What is the direction of the anal canal?
Ans: Directed downwards and backwards.

Q: What is the level of the anorectal junction?
Ans: It lies at the level of the pelvic diaphragm.

Q: What are the three areas on the anal canal, divided by the pectinate line and the Hilton's line?
Ans: Upper 15 mm: Above the pectinate/dentate line
Intermediate 15 mm: Between the pectinate and Hilton's line
Lower 8 mm: Anal verge.

Q: How is internal anal sphincter formed?
Ans: By thickening of the circular smooth muscle coat of the lower part of rectum.

Q: Which nerves supply the anal canal?
Ans: Superior hypogastric plexus and the pelvic splanchnic nerves.

Q: Which arteries supply the anal canal?
Ans: The following arteries supply the anal canal:
1. Superior rectal artery (branch of inferior mesenteric artery)
2. Middle rectal artery (branch of internal iliac artery)
3. Inferior rectal artery (branch of internal pudendal artery).

Q: Which nerves supply to the external anal sphincter?
Ans: Inferior rectal branch of the pudendal nerve and perineal branch of the fourth sacral nerve.

Q: Which blood vessel supply to the pelvis?
Ans: Internal iliac artery

Q: Describe the origin of pudendal nerve.
Ans: From the anterior rami of the second to fourth sacral roots.

Q: What are the contents of pudendal canal?
Ans: Pudendal nerve and internal pudendal vessels

ONE-LINER QUESTIONS

Q: What is the relationship of pudendal canal and obturator internus?
Ans: Pudendal canal runs medial to the obturator internus

Q: Define origin and end of pudendal canal.
Ans: *Begins*: At the posterior border of the ischiorectal fossa
Ends: At the posterior edge of the urogenital diaphragm.

Q: What are branches of pudendal nerve?
Ans: Three branches: (1) the dorsal nerve of the clitoris; (2) the inferior haemorrhoidal/rectal nerve; and (3) the perineal nerves.

Q: When is desire for micturition felt?
Ans: When the bladder contains about 300 mL of urine.

Q: What is the maximum capacity of the urinary bladder?
Ans: 500 mL

Q: Where does urinary bladder lies in an adult?
Ans: In the pelvis

Q: Where does urinary bladder lies in an infant?
Ans: Above the level of the pubic symphysis. It is an abdominal organ rather than a pelvic one.

Q: What is the embryological origin of urinary bladder?
Ans: The cloaca and mesonephric ducts.

ONE-LINER QUESTIONS
CHAPTER 2
Physiology

Q: What is the acid base abnormality in case of Conn's syndrome?
Ans: Metabolic alkalosis

Q: Where in the kidney is potassium completely reabsorbed?
Ans: Proximal convoluted tubule and distal convoluted tubule

Q: What is the cause of physiological anaemia of pregnancy?
Ans: Disproportionate increase in plasma volume

Q: Which hormone increases the excretion of calcium in kidney?
Ans: Calcitonin

Q: Which circulatory blood cell is capable of doing differentiation into plasma cells?
Ans: B lymphocytes

Q: Levels of which clotting factors remain unchanged in normal pregnancy?
Ans: Factors XI and XIII

Q: What is the major hydrogen ion buffer in urine?
Ans: Bicarbonate buffer system

Q: Which erythrocyte enzyme is responsible for CO_2 buffering?
Ans: Carbonic anhydrase

Q: Which transport mechanism is used to transfer urea from foetal circulation to maternal circulation?
Ans: Passive diffusion

Q: Where the largest volume of glucose reabsorption does occurs in the kidneys?
Ans: Proximal tubules

Q: What is the most important cation in the intracellular fluid?
Ans: Potassium

Q: Magnesium is secreted in which nephron segments?
Ans: Distal tubule

Q: By what percentage the total blood volume rises in normal pregnancy?
Ans: 40–50%

Q: Which of the following placental hormones helps to ensure adequate foetal nutrition?
Ans: Human placental lactogen

Q: In ECG lead V1 and aVR represent which portion of heart?
Ans: Right atrium and ventricle

Q: GFR is highest at which gestation period?
Ans: 16 weeks

Q: What is the change in plasma volume during pregnancy?
Ans: Increase 30–50%

Q: Glucose transported across the placenta through which mode?
Ans: Facilitated diffusion

Q: Which cancer is associated with SIADH?
Ans: Bronchial cancer

Q: What are the possible electrolyte disturbances that can occur in a new born who is diagnosed as pyloric stenosis?
Ans: Low chloride ions (Cl^-), hypokalaemia (low K^+ levels), alkalosis

Q: What percentage of total body water is intracellular?
Ans: 66%

Q: What type of compound is Beta hCG?
Ans: Glycoprotein

ONE-LINER QUESTIONS

Q: What is the volume for total blood volume that rises in normal pregnancy?
Ans: 100 mL/kg

Q: What substance in the cervical secretions attacks the bacterial lipoprotein?
Ans: Lysozyme

Q: Which cardiac condition is associated with saddle shaped ST elevation?
Ans: Pericarditis

Q: Which granulated white blood cell (WBC) has phagocytic action but constitutes only 2–3% of total WBC count?
Ans: Eosinophils

Q: What would be the diagnosis for a patient with primary infertility, 3-month amenorrhoea, elevated follicle stimulating hormone (FSH) and prolactin and beta-human chorionic gonadotropin (BHCG) positive?
Ans: Pregnancy

Q: When does β-hCG in pregnancy would be at peak?
Ans: 8–12 weeks

Q: Which is the major phospholipid constituting amniotic fluid?
Ans: Dipalmitoylphosphatidylcholine

Q: Where in the kidney is the majority of bicarbonate reabsorbed?
Ans: Proximal convoluted tubule (PCT)

Q: Closure of ductus arteriosus following lung inflation shortly after birth is mediated by which vasoactive substance?
Ans: Bradykinin

Q: Which hormone maintains the corpus luteum during the initial stage of pregnancy?
Ans: Human chorionic gonadotropin (hCG)

Q: From which part of the renal tubule does aldosterone reabsorb sodium?
Ans: Distal convoluted tubule

Q: Which is the important cation in extracellular fluid?
Ans: Sodium (Na^+)

Q: What is the volume of blood in a human body?
Ans: About 7% of body weight

Q: What is liquid portion in blood known as?
Ans: Plasma

Q: What is formula for calculating blood volume?
Ans: BV=PV/1−HC
(where BV=blood volume; PV=plasma volume; HC=haematocrit)

Q: What is shape of red blood cell?
Ans: Disc-shaped and biconcave

Q: What is another name of red blood cells?
Ans: Erythrocytes

Q: Name the enzyme which catalyses the combination of H_2O with CO_2 to produce carbonic acid (H_2CO_3).
Ans: Carbonic anhydrase

Q: What is shape of white blood cell?
Ans: Irregular

Q: Which blood vessels are responsible for the major part of blood viscosity?
Ans: Erythrocytes

Q: By which process the energy in the RBCs is produced?
Ans: Glycolytic process.

Q: Which is the most immature circulating RBCs?

ONE-LINER QUESTIONS

Ans: Reticulocytes

Q: Which blood element is most frequently used for transfusion and why?
Ans: RBCs because transfusion of RBCs increases the amount of oxygen that can be carried to the tissues of the body.

Q: Where does the breakdown of erythrocytes takes place?
Ans: Reticuloendothelial system

Q: Name the components in to which haemoglobin is degraded at the time of erythrocyte breakdown?
Ans: Iron, globin and porphyrin as well as bilirubin.

Q: Define Haematocrit or the packed cell volume (PCV).
Ans: The volume percentage of red blood cells in blood.

Q: How is haematocrit obtained?
Ans: Centrifugation of blood

Q: What is the composition of plasma and red blood cells in total blood?
Ans: Plasma 55% and red blood cells 45%.

Q: What does yellow appearance of centrifuged blood indicates?
Ans: Jaundice

Q: What does greatly thickened buffy coat appearance of centrifuged blood indicates?
Ans: Leukaemia

Q: Why does haematocrit falls in cases of macrocytic megaloblastic anaemia such as pernicious (B12 deficiency) anaemia?
Ans: Because though individual RBCs are large, total red cell mass is decreased.

Q: Define Erythrocyte sedimentation rate.
Ans: The rate at which the red blood cells sediment in 1 hour.

Q: What is the measurement unit of ESR?
Ans: mm/hour

Q: Enumerate the factors which increase ESR.
Ans: Increased amounts of proteins; large cells; lower amount of cells; inflammatory disease processes (malignancy—myeloma, systemic lupus erythematosus, polymyalgia rheumatic, and rheumatoid arthritis); and increasing age.

Q: Name the factors which decrease ESR.
Ans: Polycythaemia vera; microcytosis (haemoglobin disease, iron deficiency); dysfibrinogenaemia; hypogammaglobulinaemia; low-molecular-weight dextran; secondary conditions, which feature abnormal red blood cells (sickle cell anaemia, hereditary spherocytosis, acanthocytosis); excessive anticoagulation; hypofibrinogenaemia (disseminated intravascular coagulation, massive hepatic necrosis); cachexia; high white blood cell count; and heart failure.

Q: Which blood component is non-nucleated?
Ans: Red blood cell

Q: What is lifespan of red blood cell?
Ans: 120 days

Q: What is lifespan of white blood cell?
Ans: 12 hours to 15 days

Q: What are the types of WBC?
Ans: Granulocytes (which have granules)—Neutrophils, basophils, eosinophils.
Agranulocytes (which do not have granules)—Monocytes, and lymphocytes

Q: Which are the most common leucocytes in normal blood?
Ans: Neutrophil granulocytes

Q: What are neutrophil granulocytes also known as?

ONE-LINER QUESTIONS

Ans: Polymorphs

Q: What is the relation between number of lobes in the nucleus of WBC and the age of WBC?
Ans: The nucleus is not lobed in younger cells. Older neutrophils may have 2 to 5 lobes in their nucleus.

Q: What is the colour of coarse granules in the cytoplasm of basophils when stained with methylene blue?
Ans: Purple-blue

Q: Name the anti-coagulant and vasodilator present in basophils.
Ans: Anti-coagulant—heparin and vasodilator—histamine

Q: What is the shape of nucleus in Eosinophils?
Ans: Bilobed and spectacle-shaped

Q: Which blood component increases in parasitic infections and allergic conditions?
Ans: Eosinophils

Q: Which blood component releases leukotrienes and cytokines?
Ans: Eosinophils

Q: Name cytokines particularly released by eosinophils.
Ans: Interleukin-4 and platelet-activating factor (PAF)

Q: Where does monocytes originate?
Ans: From stem cells in bone marrow

Q: What is the half-life of monocytes in blood and tissues?
Ans: *In blood*: approximately 72 hours
In tissues: Unknown (maybe 3 months)

Q: Which blood component is the largest amongst leucocytes and what is its diameter?
Ans: Monocytes having a diameter varying between 14 μ and 18 μ.

Q: What is the shape of nucleus of monocytes?
Ans: Nucleus is round, oval, horseshoe-shaped, bean-shaped or kidney-shaped.

Q: How are lymphocytes divided depending upon the function?
Ans: Into two types: T lymphocytes B lymphocytes

Q: Which lymphocyte is concerned with cellular immunity?
Ans: T lymphocytes

Q: Which lymphocyte is concerned with humoral immunity?
Ans: B lymphocytes (due to production of immunoglobulins)

Q: Which lymphocyte comprise majority of circulating lymphocytes in plasma?
Ans: T lymphocytes

Q: Name the two types of granules present in cytoplasm of platelets.
Ans: Alpha granules and the dense granules.

Q: What is the impact of Aspirin on the cascade of coagulation?
Ans: No impact. It just causes a decline in the platelet count.

Q: Which substances are present in alpha granules of platelet?
Ans: Clotting factors: Fibrinogen, factors V and XIII
Platelet-derived growth factor
Vascular endothelial growth factor
Basic fibroblast growth factor
Endostatin
Thrombospondin

Q: Why there is an increase in the number of platelets after injury and surgery?
Ans: Because this increases the tendency of blood to clot.

Q: What is the Normal platelet count?
Ans: Between 200,000 and 400,000/mm^3.

Q: Which factor is responsible for the onset of blood clotting?

ONE-LINER QUESTIONS

Ans: Intrinsic prothrombin activator

Q: How many clotting factors are present?
Ans: Thirteen (factors I to XIII)

Q: What are the stages of blood clotting?
Ans: Three stages of blood clotting are as follows:
1. Formation/activation of prothrombin activator
2. Conversion of prothrombin into thrombin
3. Conversion of fibrinogen into fibrin

Q: What is the upper limit of the normal "bleeding time"?
Ans: About 5 minutes

Q: What is the platelet count in case of serious bleeding?
Ans: Below $20-40 \times 10^9$ per litre

Q: In which condition clotting time is prolonged?
Ans: Haemophilia

Q: What are the causes of prolonged PT?
Ans: Warfarin therapy, liver diseases (e.g. cirrhosis), disseminated intravascular coagulation (DIC), and unfractionated heparin (not low molecular weight).

Q: Which vitamin is used therapeutically if the PT is prolonged or the international normalised ratio (INR) is very high?
Ans: Vitamin K because it helps in restoring a normal prothrombin time.

Q: Mention the cases in which APTT is prolonged?
Ans: In cases of heparin or warfarin therapy and deficiency or inhibition of factors II, V, VIII, IX, X, XI, and XII.

Q: Haemophilia A is caused due to deficiency of which clotting factor?
Ans: Haemophilia A is recessive abnormality of the X chromosome and is associated with the deficiency of factor VIII.

Q: Define five categories of extracellular fluid.
Ans: (1) Interstitial fluid and lymph; (2) plasma; (3) fluid in bones; (4) fluid in dense connective tissues like cartilage; and (5) transcellular fluid (includes synovial fluid in joints, cerebrospinal fluid, intraocular fluid, digestive juices, intrapleural fluid, and pericardial fluid and peritoneal fluid, and fluid in urinary tract.

Q: In a normal woman, what is volume of plasma and its pH?
Ans: Plasma volume is about 2.5–3 L and its pH is 7.4.

Q: What are the major osmotic components of plasma?
Ans: Cations, sodium and potassium and their accompanying anions along with glucose and urea.

Q: Up to which level osmolarity can fall during pregnancy?
Ans: At least 290 mOsmol/L

Q: Name the process through which soluble drugs, e.g. propranolol can cross the lipids of blood-brain-barrier or the placenta.
Ans: By non-ionised diffusion.

Q: Give an example of facilitated transport.
Ans: Uptake of glucose by the muscle cells facilitated by insulin.

Q: What is the pH of the arterial blood?
Ans: Between 7.36 and 7.44.

Q: Why is pH of urine acidic?
Ans: pH of the urine is acidic because the normal diet leaves acidic, rather than alkaline, residues.

Q: Which is the equation for deriving the pH of ECF by measuring the concentration of bicarbonate ions (HCO_3^-) and the CO_2 dissolved in the fluid?
Ans: Henderson-Hasselbalch equation

Q: Define three different mechanisms for regulating the acid-base status.

ONE-LINER QUESTIONS

Ans: Three different mechanisms for regulating the acid-base status include the following:
1. Acid-base buffer system (which binds free H⁺)
2. Respiratory mechanism (which eliminates CO_2)
3. Renal mechanism (which excretes H+ and conserves the bases, HCO_3^-)

Q: Which mechanism is the most powerful amongst the three compensatory mechanisms?
Ans: The renal mechanism. It helps in maintaining the acid-base balance of the body fluids.

Q: Which of the following substances occur in lower concentration in foetal blood in comparison to the maternal blood?
Ans: Glucose

Q: Which buffer system plays an important role in maintaining the pH of body fluids?
Ans: Bicarbonate buffer system.

Q: Mention the conditions in which normal concentration of bicarbonate is decreased.
Ans: Renal failure (acidosis) and severe diarrhoea.

Q: What is the anion gap?
Ans: Difference between concentrations of unmeasured anions and unmeasured cations is known as the anion gap. It is calculated using the formula:
Anion gap = $[Na^+] - [HCO_3^-] - [Cl^-]$

Q: Which are the measured anions and cations in Anion gap?
Ans: The anions, which are measured, are chloride (100 mEq/L) and bicarbonate (24 mEq/L) ions. The cation, which is measured, is sodium (136 mEq/L).

Q: Which are the unmeasured anions and cations in Anion gap?
Ans: *Unmeasured cations*: Potassium, calcium, and magnesium.
Unmeasured anions: Phosphate, sulphate, proteins in anionic form

(such as albumin), and other organic anions like lactate.

Q: What are the cases in which anion gap is reduced?
Ans: Bromide poisoning and multiple myeloma.

Q: Name the two main mechanisms in which acidosis is produced.
Ans: Two main mechanisms by which acidosis is produced are as follows:
1. Increase in partial pressure of CO_2 in the body fluids (particularly in arterial blood)
2. Decrease in HCO_3^- concentration

Q: What are the values of pH and pCO_2 in respiratory acidosis?
Ans: pH <7.36 and pCO_2 >44

Q: Name the conditions associated with respiratory acidosis.
Ans: Cerebrovascular accident affecting medulla oblongata, breath holding, excessive sedation, respiratory tract obstruction, and obstructive airway disease.

Q: What are the metabolic disturbances?
Ans: Disturbances in acid-base status produced by the change in HCO_3^- concentration.

Q: Which type of acidosis is caused by uraemia?
Ans: Metabolic acidosis

Q: Which diuretic drug causes metabolic acidosis and how?
Ans: Acetazolamide. It inhibits ammonia formation within the kidneys, thereby causing metabolic acidosis.

Q: What are the causes producing alkalosis?
Ans: The following conditions can cause alkalosis:
- Decrease in partial pressure of CO_2 in the arterial blood
- Increase in HCO_3^- concentration

Q: What is the commonest clinical presentation of respiratory alkalosis?

ONE-LINER QUESTIONS

Ans: Anxiety (due to an acute fall in the concentration of H^+ ions), paraesthesiae, tetany, etc.

Q: Which type of acidosis is caused by vomiting of contents from the lower gastrointestinal tract and how?
Ans: Metabolic alkalosis. There is a loss of chloride ions and an increase in bicarbonate ions in the ECF.

Q: What are the causes of hyponatraemia?
Ans: the causes of hyponatraemia are as follows:
1. Hypothyroidism
2. Syndrome of inappropriate antidiuretic hormone or SIADH (as in subarachnoid haemorrhage and pneumonia)
3. Addison's disease
4. Liver disease
5. Diuretic therapy
6. Congestive cardiac failure
7. Bronchial carcinoma with SIADH

Q: In which cases of hyponatraemia, hypovolaemia is also caused?
Ans: Diarrhoea, vomiting, diuretics, renal tubular dysfunction, Addison's disease, etc.

Q: Name the conditions associated with hypernatraemia.
Ans: Cushing's syndrome; Conn's syndrome; diabetes insipidus along with steroid therapy and the administration of hypertonic saline.

Q: Name the drugs causing hypokalaemia.
Ans: Salbutamol; vitamin B12; carbenoxolone; liquorice; and bendroflumethiazide.

Q: What are the causes of hyperkalaemia?
Ans: Type IV renal tubular acidosis; hyperparathyroidism; hypoadrenalism; CAH; Addison's disease; angiotensin-converting enzyme (ACE) inhibitors; and rhabdomyolysis.

Q: What are the conditions associated with hypocalcaemia?

Ans: Convulsions, papilloedema, psychosis, muscle cramps, spasm, and tetany.

Q: Which lung volume signifies the normal depth of breathing?
Ans: Tidal volume.

Q: What are the normal values of tidal volume, inspiratory reserve volume, expiratory reserve volume, and residual volume.
Ans: Tidal volume, 500 mL; inspiratory reserve volume, 3,300 mL; expiratory reserve volume, 1,000 mL; and residual volume, 1–1.5 L.

Q: What technique is used to measure residual volume?
Ans: Indirectly by a dilution technique

Q: What is Inspiratory capacity? What is its normal value?
Ans: It is the maximum volume of air that is inspired after normal expiration. It includes tidal volume and IRV. Its normal value is 3,800 mL.

Q: How does FEV1 varies with age?
Ans: The normal value of FEV1 in an adult patient is about 85% at the age of 20 years, falling to about 70% at the age of 60–70 years.

Q: What are the two main components of the pulmonary function test of respiratory disease?
Ans: Forced expiratory volume in the first second (FEV1), and forced vital capacity (FVC)

Q: Describe how forced expiratory volume in one second (FEV1) and forced vital capacity (FVC) are affected in restrictive lung disease.
Ans: Both are reduced. However, the decline in FVC is more than that of FEV1, resulting in a ratio of FEV1/FVC which is usually higher than 80%.

Q: Describe how restrictive and obstructive respiratory disease are characterised by difficulty in inspiration/expiration.
Ans: *Restrictive respiratory disease*: Abnormal respiratory condition characterised by difficulty in inspiration.

ONE-LINER QUESTIONS

Obstructive respiratory disease: Abnormal respiratory condition characterised by difficulty in expiration.

Q: Where are the primary centres for the control of respiration situated?
Ans: In the medulla and pons of the brainstem

Q: Diaphragm is driven by the activity of which nerve?
Ans: Phrenic nerve (C3–C5)

Q: What is the source of the most important stimulation for the respiratory centre?
Ans: Input comes from the chemoreceptors:
1. *Central chemoreceptors*: On the surface of upper medulla (but separate from the medullary respiratory centres)]
2. *Peripheral chemoreceptors*: Around the aortic arch and the carotid body.

Q: Which is the only respiratory stimulant used in clinical practice and why?
Ans: Doxapram because it does not cause other stimulatory side effects (e.g. risk of convulsions).

Q: What is Hering-Bruer reflex?
Ans: It is a mechanism contributing to the cessation of inspiration and initiation of expiration, triggered as a method for preventing the overinflation of lungs.

Q: What is normal value of minute ventilation in adults?
Ans: 5–8 L/minute

Q: Mention two components of dead space.
Ans: Two components of dead space are as follows:
1. *Anatomical dead space*: Total volume of air present in the conducting zone (i.e. the conducting bronchioles and above), where no gaseous exchange can occur
2. *Alveolar dead space*: Volume of air present in the respiratory zone

(i.e. respiratory bronchioles and below)

Q: Define relation between the compliance of lungs and volume as well as pressure.
Ans: Compliance of lungs and chest wall is expressed as volume change per unit change in pressure

Q: How many factors are responsible for the collapsing tendency of lungs? Name them.
Ans: Two factors, namely elastic property of lung tissues and the surface tension

Q: Which are the factors, which save the lungs from collapsing?
Ans: Negative intrapleural pressure and the presence of surfactant.

Q: Which factors lead to respiratory distress syndrome?
Ans: Lack of surfactant and lung immaturity.

Q: Which drug may be beneficial in cases where there is a risk of delivery before 34 weeks of gestation due to respiratory distress?
Ans: Intramuscular injection of dexamethasone and betamethasone

Q: In which forms, transportation of oxygen takes place from alveoli to the tissues?
Ans: 3% of total oxygen is transported in its physical form by dissolving in the water of plasma. Transportation of oxygen in combination with haemoglobin as oxyhaemoglobin accounts for rest 97% of oxygen.

Q: What is the shape of oxygen dissociation curve and why?
Ans: The shape of oxygen dissociation curve is sigmoid-shaped (not hyperbolic) because of the increasing affinity of haemoglobin for successive oxygen molecules after binding to the first one.

Q: What are the factors which shift the ODC to the right?
Ans: Haemoglobin S; increased red cell concentration of 2, 3 diphosphoglycerate (2, 3 DPG); anaemia and heart failure; and situations include high temperature, low oxygen and high pCO_2 levels.

ONE-LINER QUESTIONS

Q: What is Haldane's effect?
Ans: Increased concentration of carbon dioxide will displace oxygen from haemoglobin and binding of oxygen to haemoglobin will displace carbon dioxide from the blood.

Q. What is Bohr's effect?
Ans. The affinity of oxygen to bind with haemoglobin is inversely related both to the acidity and the concentration of carbon dioxide.

Q: What is the role of 2,3-DPG on ODC?
Ans: Higher levels of 2,3-DPG shift the ODC curve to the right, whereas low levels of 2,3-DPG cause a leftward shift.

Q: What is the value of normal ventilation/perfusion ratio? When does this increases and why?
Ans: Normal value is 0.8. It exceeds 1.0. It exceeds during maximal exercise because during maximal exercise, alveolar ventilation may rise to about 80 L/min, while alveolar perfusion rises to about 25 L/min.

Q: Which is the method assessing arterial oxygen saturation and heart rate?
Ans: Pulse oximetry

Q: When does cyanosis occurs?
Ans: It occurs when arterial blood contains more than 5 g/dL reduced haemoglobin.

Q: What leads to retention of mucous secretions during anaesthesia?
Ans: Cough reflex is depressed during anaesthesia, which leads to retention of mucous secretions.

Q: What is end-diastolic volume?
Ans: The point at which the maximum ventricular volume has been reached.

Q: What leads to first heart sound "lub"?

Ans: The closure of atrioventricular valves (both the mitral valve on the left side and tricuspid valve on the right side) is heard as the first heart sound, "lub".

Q: What leads to second heart sound "dub"?
Ans: The reduction in ventricular pressure leads to the aortic and pulmonary valves to close. This is heard as the second heart sound, "dub".

Q: How is first heart sound different from second heart sound?
Ans: The second heart sound is about 20% shorter than the first sound. It is higher in frequency, i.e. about 50 Hz compared with 35 Hz for the first sound.

Q: In which cases third heart sound can occur?
Ans: Mitral and tricuspid regurgitation, constrictive pericarditis, dilated left ventricle, and acute myocardial infarction

Q: When does fourth heart sound occurs?
Ans: Fourth heart sound (always pathological) occurs during atrial contractions (when a jet of blood hits an excessively stiff ventricle).

Q: What are normal values of PR and QT interval?
Ans: Normal PR interval lies between 0.1 and 0.2 seconds and normal QT interval varies between 0.3 and 0.4 seconds

Q: In which cases QT interval is increased?
Ans: Hypocalcaemia, hypokalaemia, rheumatic carditis, and medication with quinidine.

Q: What are ECG changes in sub-endocardial MI?
Ans: Sub-endocardial MI is associated with segment ST depression (not elevation) and T wave inversion in leads facing the infarction.

Q: Where does the origin of the cardiac impulse starts at the sinoatrial node?
Ans: At the sinoatrial node

Q: What is the relation between arterial blood pressure and

elasticity and the diameter of blood vessel?
Ans: It is indirectly proportional to elasticity and the diameter of blood vessel.

Q: How are Korotkoff sounds produced?
Ans: These are produced locally by the turbulence of blood being forced past the narrow segment of a partially occluded artery.

Q: What are the contents of glomerulus?
Ans: Glomerulus consists of a tuft of capillaries enclosed by Bowman capsule. There are glomerular capillaries interposed between afferent arteriole on one end and efferent arteriole on the other end.

Q: What structures are present in Loop of Henle?
Ans: It consists of the thin descending limb, hairpin bend, and a thick ascending limb.

Q: Name the processes involved in urine formation.
Ans: Three processes: glomerular filtration, tubular reabsorption, and tubular secretion.

Q: What is glomerular filtrate?
Ans: When blood passes through glomerular capillaries, the plasma is filtered into the Bowman capsule. All the substances of plasma are filtered except the plasma proteins. The filtered fluid is called glomerular filtrate.

Q: What are the substances reabsorbed from the various parts of the nephron?
Ans: The following substances are reabsorbed from various parts of nephron:
Proximal convoluted tubule: About 88% of the filtrate is reabsorbed in PCT. Other substances reabsorbed proximal are glucose, amino acids, sodium, potassium, calcium, bicarbonates, chlorides, phosphates, urea, uric acid and water.
Loop of Henle: Sodium and chloride
Distal convoluted tubule: Sodium, calcium, bicarbonate, and water

Q: Which substances are secreted in which segments of renal tubules?
Ans: The following substances are secreted in which segments of renal tubules:
1. Potassium in proximal and distal convoluted tubules and collecting ducts
2. Ammonia is in the proximal convoluted tubule
3. Hydrogen ions in the proximal and distal convoluted tubules
4. Maximum hydrogen ion in proximal tubule
5. Urea in loop of Henle.

Q: What factors are required to determine the plasma clearance of a particular substance?
Ans: Volume of urine excreted; concentration of the substance in urine; and concentration of the substance in blood.

Q How is clearance calculated?
Ans. Clearance is calculated using the following formula: $C=UV/P$, Where, C = clearance; U = concentration of the substance in urine; V = volume of urine flow; P = concentration of the substance in plasma.

Q: What is normal GFR of both the kidneys?
Ans: 120 mL/minute.

Q: Which is an accessory digestive organ?
Ans: Pancreas

Q: What is the main function of Saliva?
Ans: It is required for normal speech. It is also required for antisepsis in the mouth and taste sensation.

Q: What is the composition of gastric juice?
Ans: gastric juice is composed of the following components:
1. Enzymes: Pepsin, rennin, gastric lipase, gelatinase, urease, etc.
2. Inorganic substances: Hydrochloric acid, sodium, calcium, potassium, bicarbonate, chloride, phosphate, etc.
3. Organic substances: Mucus and intrinsic factor.

Q: What are the functions of HCl in the stomach?

ONE-LINER QUESTIONS

Ans: HCL performs the following functions:
Activates pepsinogen into pepsin
Bacteriolytic action: Killing some of the bacteria entering the stomach along with the food substances
Provides of acidic medium, which is necessary for the action of various enzymes.

Q: What are the functions of pancreas?
Ans: *Endocrine function*: Production of hormones.
Exocrine function: Secretion of digestive juice called pancreatic juice.

Q: Name the hormones stimulating pancreatic secretion.
Ans: Secretin and cholecystokinin

Q: What are functions performed by the liver?
Ans: The liver performs the following functions:
Maintenance of the blood glucose levels: When there is a decline in the blood glucose levels, liver glycogen is broken down to form glucose. On the other hand, when there is an increase in blood glucose levels, the excessive glucose is converted by the liver into glycogen.
Deamination of amino acids: NH_4 ions are toxic and are converted into urea and excreted in the urine.
Synthesis of 25-hydroxycholecalciferol
Manufacture of plasma proteins
Inactivation of steroid hormones

Q: What is of liver function test?
Ans: It include estimation of: bilirubin (direct and indirect); prothrombin time; serum albumin levels; and estimation of the levels of hepatic enzymes: transaminases (AST, aspartate transaminase or SGOT and ALT, alanine transaminase or SGPT), alkaline phosphatase, and g-glutamyl transpeptidase.

Q: What causes kernicterus in a newborn child?
Ans: The blood-brain barrier (BBB) may not be mature enough in a newborn child, thereby allowing excessive bilirubin to pass through resulting in the development of kernicterus.

Q: What are the symptoms of portal hypertension?
Ans: Ascites, hepatic encephalopathy; and development of varices at the porto-caval anastomosis.

Q: What are the consequences of removal of gall bladder?
Ans: Loss of bile (resulting in poor digestion and impaired absorption of the meal). Hence, there may be abdominal discomfort, following a fatty meal.

Q: What are the hormones secreted by placenta?
Ans: It synthesizes and secretes the hormones—progestins and oestrogens, chorionic gonadotropins, relaxin and placental lactogens.

Q: What is half-life of hCG and LH?
Ans: hCG: 24 hours; LH:2 hours

Q: What are the major functions of hPL?
Ans: the major functions of hPL include the following:
1. Helps in regulating the mother's metabolism during pregnancy.
2. hPL ensures that there is adequate amount of nutrient supply for the foetus by helping in movement of nutrients across the placenta.

Q: When are higher levels of relaxin present in pregnancy?
Ans: Higher levels are present early in pregnancy.

Q: What is the role of placenta in maintaining immunity?
Ans: Placenta maintains foetal maternal immunological balance—passive immunity and suppression of the mother's immune response against the foetus (immunosuppression).

Q: Which immunoglobulin is the major type of antibodies that is able to cross the placental barrier?
Ans: IgG.

Q: What is Chadwick's or Jacquemier's sign? When is this observed during gestation?
Ans: The vaginal walls show a bluish discolouration as the pelvic

blood vessels become congested. This sign can be observed by 8–10 weeks of gestation.

Q: What is Osiander's sign? When is this observed during gestation?
Ans: There is increased pulsation in the vagina felt through the lateral vaginal fornix at 8 weeks of gestation.

Q: Name three layers in which the uterine musculature during pregnancy is arranged?
Ans: The three layers in which the uterine musculature during pregnancy is arranged include the following:
1. An outer hood-like layer arching over the fundus and extending into the various ligaments
2. Middle layer composed of dense network of muscle fibres perforated in all directions by the blood vessels
3. An inner layer comprising of sphincter-like fibres around the orifices of fallopian tube and internal os of the cervix.

Q: How are muscle fibres in the middle layer of the uterine musculature during pregnancy are arranged?
Ans: They are arranged in an interlacing, "figure of 8" manner with blood vessels lying between these fibres.

Q: What is weight of uterus at term?
Ans: Approximately 1,100 grams at term.

Q: What is Palmer sign?
Ans: Sensing of uterine contractions during bimanual examination by the examiner is described as Palmer sign.

Q: When can Palmer's sign be felt?
Ans: 4–8 weeks of gestation.

Q: What is difference between uterine soufflé and foetal soufflé?
Ans: *Uterine soufflé*: This is a soft blowing sound synchronous with the maternal pulse. It is caused by rush of blood through the uterine arteries.
Foetal soufflé: It is a sharp whistling sound synchronous with the

foetal pulse. It is caused by the rush of blood through the umbilical arteries.

Q: What is Godell's sign?
Ans. Godell's sign can be described as the softening of the vaginal portion of the cervix resulting due to increased vascularization, which is the result of hypertrophy and engorgement of the vessels below the enlarging uterus.

Q: At what gestational age Godell's sign becomes evident?
Ans: By 6 weeks of pregnancy.

Q: What is the concentration of total plasma proteins at term?
Ans: 230 grams at term.

Q: What is the average haemoglobin concentration at term?
Ans: 12.5 g/dL.

Q: What is the total amount of iron transferred to placenta and cord?
Ans: 90 mg.

Q: What is the total iron requirement during pregnancy?
Ans: 600–700 mg (6–7 mg of daily requirement of elemental iron for about 100 days).

Q: What is normal value of aspartate aminotransferase (IU/L) during pregnancy?
Ans: 10–30 IU/L

Q: What is normal value of bilirubin (μmol/L) during pregnancy??
Ans: 3–16

Q: How does sensitivity to insulin vary during pregnancy?
Ans: *First half of pregnancy*: There is an increased sensitivity to insulin.
Second half of pregnancy (especially after 24 weeks of gestation): Development of insulin resistance.

Q: Which hormones are increased during pregnancy?

Ans: Sex hormone-binding globulin (b-hCG); prolactin; total thyroxin (as there is an increase in the binding proteins); oestrogens; Beta human chorionic gonadotropin (b-hCG); and progestogens

ONE-LINER QUESTIONS
CHAPTER 3
Biochemistry

Q: What kind of change occurs in glucose-controlling hormone in the body after consumption of protein-rich meal?
Ans: Insulin increases glucagon decreases

Q: Which processes occur exclusively in mitochondria?
Ans: Oxidative phosphorylation, Kreb's cycle, and electron transport chain

Q: Which test increases the number of copies of DNA?
Ans: Polymerase chain reaction (PCR)

Q: What mechanism is required for myometrial contraction?
Ans: Electron transport chain

Q: Which step occurs in the mitochondria releasing ATP?
Ans: Oxidative phosphorylation

Q: At which phase of the cell cycle does DNA replication occur?
Ans: S phase (synthesis phase)

Q: What is the most expected risk for a patient who is *BRCA1* positive?
Ans: Breast cancer

Q: What is the active form of vitamin D?
Ans: Calcitriol (1, 25-$(OH)_2D_3$)

Q: What is the major role of glucocorticoids in glucose metabolism?
Ans: Gluconeogenesis

Q: What type of compound is histones?
Ans: Protein

Q: What is the pathophysiology that explains that vitamin A can cause birth defects in the child during pregnancy?
Ans: Hyper-vitaminosis A

Q: Where does fatty acid synthesis occur within the cell?
Ans: Cytosol

Q: What is the function of the enzyme glucose-6-phosphatase in carbohydrate metabolism?
Ans: Conversion glucose-6-phosphate to glucose

Q: What is the parent compound from which most eicosanoids are derived?
Ans: Arachidonic acids

Q: Which process occurs in the mitochondria where uses electrons transport to generate adenosine triphosphate (ATP)?
Ans: Oxidative phosphorylation

Q: Which biochemical technique is used for prenatal identification of cystic fibrosis by using specifically amplifying predetermined DNA sequences?
Ans: Polymerase chain reaction

Q: Where does urea cycle occur?
Ans: Liver

Q: What is the active form of vitamin D?
Ans: 1,25-dihydroxycholecalciferol

Q: Glycolysis takes place in which part of the cell?
Ans: Cytoplasm

Q: Which cellular organelle is especially abundant in cells that synthesize antibodies?
Ans: Rough endoplasmic reticulum

Q: Glucagon works by which mechanism to reverse the hypoglycaemia?

ONE-LINER QUESTIONS

Ans: Gluconeogenesis

Q: Which of the following laboratory techniques is used for RNA analysis?
Ans: Northern blotting

Q: Which protein is coiled in DNA?
Ans: Histones

Q: What is the action of vitamin C?
Ans: Synthesize collagen

Q: What is the primary function of DNA polymerase?
Ans: Addition of nucleotides

Q: Which technique is used for the detection of protein?
Ans: Western blotting

Q: Which nucleotide is only present in DNA?
Ans: Thymine

Q: What is the most abundant carbohydrate in the breast milk?
Ans: Lactose

Q: Which amino acid liberates nitric oxide (NO)?
Ans: L-arginine

Q: Cristae are present in which cell organelle?
Ans: Mitochondria

Q: What is another name of cell membrane? What are its functions?
Ans: It is known as plasma membrane or plasmalemma.
Functions: 1. Separates the fluid outside the cell called extracellular fluid (ECF) from the fluid inside the cell called intracellular fluid (ICF).
2. Controls the intracellular electrolyte and biochemical environment.

3. Provides adhesion between individual cells and bears the individual's major human leucocyte antigens (HLA).

Q: Name two zones of cytoplasm.
Ans: 1. Ectoplasm (peripheral part of cytoplasm, situated just beneath the cell membrane)
2. Endoplasm (inner part of cytoplasm, placed between the ectoplasm and the nucleus)

Q: Name the cytoplasmic *organelles without limiting membrane.*
Ans: Ribosomes and cytoskeleton

Q: What is the thickness of the cell membrane?
Ans: It varies from 75Å to 111Å.

Q: Which organelle forms a link between nucleus and cell membrane?
Ans: Endoplasmic reticulum

Q: What is the function of RER?
Ans: 1. Synthesis of proteins (which are subsequently secreted outside the cell)
2. Degradation of worn-out cytoplasmic organelles like mitochondria

Q: What is the function of SER?
Ans: Synthesis of non-protein substances such as cholesterol and steroids

Q: What is the location of cis and trans face of Golgi apparatus?
Ans: The cis face is situated near the ER. The trans face is situated near the cell membrane.

Q: Which organelle is known as "shipping department of the cell" and why?
Ans: Golgi apparatus because the major function of Golgi apparatus is processing, packing, labelling, and delivery of proteins and other molecules like lipids to different parts of the cell.

ONE-LINER QUESTIONS

Q: Which organelle is known as "garbage system" of the cell and why?
Ans: Lysosomes because of their degradation activity.

Q: What are primary and secondary lysosomes?
Ans: Primary lysosomes are pinched off from Golgi apparatus. Secondary lysosomes are the active lysosomes which are formed by the fusion of a primary lysosome with phagosome or endosome.

Q: Name the important lysosomal enzymes.
Ans: Proteases, lipases, amylases, and nucleases

Q: How do secretory lysosomes form?
Ans: Conventional lysosomes are modified into secretory lysosomes upon combination with secretory granules (which contain the particular secretory product of the cell).

Q: Define which substance is secreted by which type of lysosome.
Ans: Lysosomes in the cytotoxic T lymphocytes and natural killer cells secrete perforin and granzymes; secretory lysosomes of melanocytes secrete melanin; and secretory lysosomes of mast cells secrete serotonin.

Q: What is another name of peroxisomes? From which organelle do they originate?
Ans: Peroxisomes are also called as microbodies. These are the membrane-bound vesicles, which are pinched off from the ER.

Q: What are the main functions of peroxisomes?
Ans: The peroxisomes perform the following functions:

- The breakdown the fatty acids through beta (β)-oxidation
- Degrading the toxic substances such as hydrogen peroxide and other metabolic products in the cell
- These are the major site of oxygen utilisation in the cells
- Accelerate gluconeogenesis from fats
- Degrade purine to uric acid
- Participate in the formation of myelin

- Helps in formation of bile acids

Q: Where is the centrosome situated?
Ans: Almost in the centre of cell, close to nucleus

Q: What are centrioles? What is its size and composition?
Ans: These are two hollow cylindrical structures, which forms centrosomes. These are 0.3–0.7 µm in length and are made up of proteins.

Q: Where does the formation of secretory vesicles occur?
Ans: These are formed in the ER and processed and packed in Golgi apparatus.

Q What is shape and size of mitochondrion?
Ans: It is rod- or oval-shaped, elongated structure with a diameter of 0.5–1 µ.

Q: Name the enzymes present in outer membrane of mitochondrion.
Ans: Acetyl-CoA synthetase and glycerophosphate acetyltransferase

Q: Which components form the respiratory chain or electron transport system?
Ans: The enzymes and other protein molecules in cristae of mitochondrion form respiratory chain or electron transport system.

Q: Name the organelle which is capable of replicating itself.
Ans: Mitochondrion. It is the only organelle in the cell other than nucleus, which has its own DNA and is therefore capable of replicating itself.

Q: What is the composition of nucleus?
Ans: It is covered by a membrane called nuclear membrane and contains many components, i.e. nucleoplasm, chromatin, and the nucleolus.

Q: What is chromatin?

ONE-LINER QUESTIONS

Ans It is a thread-like material made up of large molecules of DNA, which are compactly packed with the help of a specialized basic protein called histone, hence forming a DNA-histone complex.

Q: Which organelle contains a complete blueprint of all the hereditary characteristics of that species?
Ans: Chromosome

Q: What are the functions of nucleus?
Ans:
- Controlling metabolism, protein synthesis, cell growth, and division
- Synthesis of RNA and formation of ribosomal subunits
- Nuclear RNA is a precursor of cytoplasmic ribosomal RNA. It also sends genetic instruction to the cytoplasm for protein synthesis through messenger RNA (mRNA).
- Nucleus controls the division of cells through genes and transformation of genetic information from one generation of the species to the next

Q: What is the size and composition of ribosomes?
Ans: Diameter 15 nm. These are made from complexes of RNAs (65%) and proteins (35%).

Q: Which cytoplasmic organelles are called "protein factories"?
Ans: Ribosomes. Because they are mainly concerned with synthesis of proteins required for intracellular metabolism.

Q: What are the functions of free ribosomes?
Ans: Synthesis of proteins in haemoglobin, peroxisome, and mitochondria

Q: Which are the three major protein components of cytoskeleton?
Ans (1) Microtubule, (2) intermediate filaments, and (3) microfilaments.

Q: Name the protein by which the microtubules are formed?

Ans: These are formed by bundles of globular protein called "tubulin", which is composed of two subunits, namely α-subunit and β-subunit.

Q: Name the subclasses of intermediate filaments.
Ans: Five subclasses: (1) keratins (in epithelial cells); (2) glial filaments (in astrocytes); (3) neurofilaments (in nerve cells); (4) vimentin (in many types of cells); and (5) desmin (in muscle fibres).

Q: What are the components of microfilaments?
Ans: These filaments are made up of non-tubular contractile proteins called actin and myosin.

Q: What forms the chemical basis of hereditary characters through the formation of genes?
Ans: Deoxyribonucleic acid (DNA)

Q: What is the composition of DNA molecule?
Ans: Each DNA molecule consists of several nucleotides each of which is composed of deoxyribose (sugar), phosphoric acid, and four types of bases.

Q: Name the organic (nitrogenous) bases present in DNA.
Ans: Purines: adenine (A) and guanine (G), and pyrimidines: thymine (T) and cytosine (C).

Q: What is the hereditary information that is encoded in DNA called?
Ans: Genome

Q: Which enzyme assists in DNA replication and how?
Ans: DNA polymerase. It initiates DNA replication by binding to a piece of single-stranded DNA.

Q: What is annealing?
Ans: Annealing is a process in which specific synthetic oligonucleotides sequences (known as primers) are bound to the complementary sequences on the target DNA. This is known as annealing.

ONE-LINER QUESTIONS

Q: What are the indications for using PCR?
Ans: 1. Useful for rapid diagnosis of conditions where traditional method of culturing the bacteria can take several weeks (such as tuberculosis)
2. Technique allows scientists directly and exponentially to amplify small samples of DNA and even RNA through reverse transcriptase PCR
3. Used for the prenatal diagnosis of conditions such as cystic fibrosis

Q: Name the enzymes, which recognise a short nucleotide sequence (restriction site) in a double-stranded DNA molecule.
Ans: Restriction endonucleases

Q: What is the principle of southern blot hybridization?
Ans: This technique involves identification of specific DNA fragments separated through electrophoresis. The individual fragments are detected through probe hybridisation.

Q: Which is the principal carbohydrate used in body metabolism?
Ans: Glucose

Q: What is transcription?
Ans: The formation of RNA is catalysed by RNA polymerase, which links together RNA nucleotides using a DNA template in a process called transcription.

Q: Which RNA carries the genetic code of the amino acid sequence for synthesis of protein from the DNA to the cytoplasm?
Ans: Messenger RNA

Q: What acts as a central compound in metabolism of carbohydrates, proteins, and fats?
Ans: Acetyl coenzyme A

Q: Name the processes by which glucose-6-phosphate can be metabolized.

Ans: It can be metabolized by the anaerobic glycolysis (Embden-Meyerhof pathway), aerobic glycolysis (Kreb's cycle), or pentose shunt.

Q: Which blood cells lack Kreb's cycle?
Ans: Erythrocytes because they have no nucleus

Q: How many molecules of ATP are produced by glycolysis of one molecule of glucose?
Ans: Two molecules of ATP

Q: Which reactions are not reversible in glycolysis?
Ans: All the reactions of glycolysis are reversible except for the reactions catalysed by hexokinase, phosphofructokinase, and pyruvate kinase.

Q: Which process forms the common pathway for the metabolism of carbohydrates, fats, and proteins?
Ans: Kreb's cycle or the citric acid cycle because it results in the complete oxidation of acetyl CoA to carbon dioxide and water.

Q: Which is the rate-limiting step in the TCA cycle? Name the enzyme involved in it.
Ans: The conversion of isocitrate to α-ketoglutarate. The enzyme involved is the citrate synthetase.

Q: Which point serves as a switch point in TCA cycle, which controls the main function of the cycle?
Ans Channelling of pyruvate into TCA cycle as acetyl CoA or as oxaloacetate serves as a switch point in TCA cycle. If pyruvate is channelled to acetyl CoA then the cycle will generate mainly energy. On the other hand, if pyruvate is channelled into oxaloacetate, then the main function of the cycle would be to produce carbon skeletons for the synthesis of amino acids or fats.

Q: Which one is more energy efficient—aerobic respiration or anaerobic respiration?
Ans: Aerobic respiration. In aerobic respiration, a single molecule of glucose produces 36 molecules of ATP. On the other hand, one

molecule of glucose undergoing anaerobic respiration produces 2 molecules of ATP.

Q: Which cycle plays a dual or amphibolic role by exhibiting a vital role in both catabolism and anabolism?
Ans: Kreb's cycle

Q: What are the components of electron transport system?
Ans: It consists of four large protein complexes and two small independent components known as ubiquinone (coenzyme Q10) and cytochrome C.

Q: Which is an alternative pathway to glycolysis and TCA cycle for the oxidation of glucose?
Ans: Hexose monophosphate (HMP) shunt

Q: Name the enzymes involved in phosphorylation of glucose to glucose-6-phosphate.
Ans: Enzyme hexokinase (in muscle) and glucokinase (in liver).

Q: What factor initiates the process of glycogenolysis and where does it occurs?
Ans: It is usually triggered by low blood glucose levels and takes place in liver and muscle.

Q: Name the enzymes involved in process of glycogenolysis.
Ans: 1. Enzyme phosphorylase [breaks only α-(1,4) linkages]
2. Debranching enzymes [breaks only α-(1,6) linkages].

Q: Which are the three hormonal activators of glycogenolysis?
Ans: (1) Glucagon; (2) adrenaline (epinephrine); and (3) cortisol.

Q: What is Cori cycle?
Ans The cyclic process by which lactic acid is converted to glucose in the liver and eventually reappears as muscle glycogen is known as Cori cycle.

Q: Which is an important pathway for supplying glucose to various tissues when glucose is not available (at the times of prolonged fasting, starvation, or strenuous exercises)?
Ans: Gluconeogenesis

Q: What are the functions of galactose?
Ans: Galactose is important for the formation of glycolipids and glycoprotein and for the formation of lactose during lactation.

Q: Which are the two routes through which fructose enter the glycolytic pathway?
Ans: 1. Liver: Most of the fructose in the body is metabolised through this pathway.
2. Muscle and adipose tissues

Q: What are the functions of galactose?
Ans: 1. It is a constituent of glycolipids (cerebrosides), chondromucoids, and mucoprotein
2. It is also required for the lactose synthesis in the mammary gland with help of the enzyme lactose synthetase.

Q: Which cells secrete glucagon?
Ans: The islets of Langerhans

Q: Which is the most common and also the first fatty acid to be synthesised in the body?
Ans: Palmitate [$CH_3(CH_2)14COOH$]

Q: What is beta-oxidation?
Ans: A process of four enzymic steps in which fatty acids are broken down in the mitochondrion to release acetyl CoA, NADH, and FADH2.

Q: Which enzyme acts in oxidation of acyl CoA to 2-enoyl CoA?
Ans: Enzyme acyl CoA dehydrogenase

Q: Define saturated fatty acids and unsaturated fatty acids.

ONE-LINER QUESTIONS

Ans: Saturated fatty acids: Have no carbon-carbon double bonds; the carbon atoms are saturated with the maximum number of hydrogen atoms.
Unsaturated fatty acids: Have one or more double bonds.

Q: Name the two main ketone bodies in the body.
Ans: Acetoacetate and β-hydroxybutyrate

Q: Which enzyme helps in formation of beta-hydroxybutyrate?
Ans: β-hydroxybutyrate dehydrogenase

Q: What are the functions of prostaglandins?
Ans: They help in stimulating many of the body's processes such as modulation of ion transport across membranes, inflammatory response, propagation of synaptic transmission, regulation of the blood flow to specific organs, induction of sleep, etc.

Q: Name the purines and puridines.
Ans: Purines—adenine and guanine
Pyrimidines—thymine, uracil, and cytosine
Of the various pyrimidines, cytosine is found in both DNA and RNA, but thymine is only found in DNA and uracil is only found in RNA.

Q: How does concentration of uric acid varies in pregnancy.
Ans: By 8 weeks of gestation, the concentrations of uric acid decrease significantly and are maintained until about 24 weeks. After that, the concentrations increase so that by term they are greater than the prepregnancy values in the majority of patients.

Q: Which is the most important among essential amino acids?
Ans: Methionine

Q: By which process different proteins can be separated based on their pattern of charge?
Ans: Ion exchange chromatography

Q: How does Ca^{++} acts as a second messenger?
Ans:

1. Binding to an effector molecule, such as an enzyme, thereby activating it
2. Binding to an intermediary cytosolic calcium-binding protein such as calmodulin

Q: How does concentration of nitric oxide varies in pregnancy?
Ans: NO production is increased in normal and even more so in abnormal pregnancies.

Q: Which vitamin is involved in the tricarboxylic acid (Kreb's) cycle?
Ans: Folic acid

Q: Which vitamin is essential for the metabolism of folic acid in the human?
Ans: Vitamin B12

Q: Sprue is caused by deficiency of which vitamin?
Ans: Folates

Q: Excess of which vitamin lead to the formation of oxalate stones in the urinary tract?
Ans: Vitamin C

ONE-LINER QUESTIONS
CHAPTER 4
Pathology

Q: Which cancer is associated with endometrioma?
Ans: Clear cell carcinoma (uterine)

Q: How much percentage do HPV 16 and HPV 18 contribute to the cases of cervical cancer?
Ans: 70%

Q: What is the management of choice in a pregnant woman suspected to have pulmonary embolism?
Ans: Ventilation scan should be done.

Q: Which hormone is insensitive to NSAIDs and a potent inflammatory mediator?
Ans: Bradykinin

Q: What is the cellular process that occurs in the breast in pregnancy which allows the woman to nurse the infant during the post-partum period?
Ans: Lobular hyperplasia

Q: What histology constitutes the majority of vulvar cancers?
Ans: Squamous cell carcinoma

Q: What are the predisposing factors for atherosclerosis?
Ans: Hyperlipidaemia, hypertriglyceridaemia, hypercholesterolaemia, hypertension, diabetes, smoking, and obesity.

Q: What are the chemical mediators involved in production of an inflammatory response?

Ans: Bradykinin, globulin permeability factor, 5-hydroxytryptamine, histamine, and plasma kinins.

Q: What is amyloidosis?
Ans: It is the deposition of "amyloid material" (complex mucopolysaccharide containing globulins) in the connective tissue stroma and the walls of blood vessels of certain tissues and organs.

Q: What may be the terminal manifestation of amyloidosis?
Ans: Renal failure may be the terminal manifestation of amyloidosis.

Q: Which is an essential feature of abscess formation?
Ans: Pyaemia

Q: What is berry aneurysm? Where is its most common occurrence?
Ans: Berry aneurysms result from abnormalities in the medial wall of the arteries. They are most often found in the circle of Willis.

Q: Which pathogen is commonly isolated from intra-abdominal pus?
Ans: Clostridia

Q: Whatmchemical substance elicits a febrile response?
Ans: Interleukin

Q: Which are the causes of generalized lymphadenopathy (LAP)?
Ans: HIV seroconversion illness; Q fever; syphilis; and *Toxoplasma gondii*

Q: Within what time from injury do macrophages replace neutrophils in case of cutaneous wound healing?
Ans: 48–96 hours

Q: What are the cell changes associated with apoptosis?
Ans: Karyorrhexis; cell shrinkage (pyknosis); nuclear shrinkage and condensation of chromatin; and formation of cytoplasmic blebs called apoptotic bodies.

Q: What are cardinal signs of inflammation?

ONE-LINER QUESTIONS

Ans: Redness, swelling, heat, pain, and loss of function.

Q: Which are the chemical mediators involved in production of an inflammatory response?
Ans: Globulin permeability factor, bradykinin, 5-hydroxytryptamine, plasma kinins, and histamine.

Q: Which is the crucial factor in formation of an inflammatory exudate?
Ans: Increased permeability of the vessel wall to plasma proteins.

Q: Name the conditions in which formation of exudate occurs.
Ans: Peritoneal malignancy, tuberculous peritonitis, Budd-Chiari syndrome, pancreatic ascites, chylous ascites, Meigs' syndrome, etc.

Q: Which is not an essential feature of abscess formation?
Ans: Pyaemia

Q: What are the general features of chronic inflammation?
Ans: Proliferation of blood vessels and fibroblasts; infiltration by mononuclear cells; tissue destruction, evidence of the repair process, characterised by migration of capillaries and fibroblasts; and formation of collagen.

Q: What is composition of granuloma?
Ans: It is composed of modified macrophages known as epithelioids cells in the centre, with some interspersed multinucleate giant cells, surrounded peripherally by lymphocytes (mainly T cells), and fibroblasts or collagen depending upon the age of granuloma.

Q: Name the steps involved in the process of repair.
Ans: It involves initial inflammatory reaction by the body; clearance by proteolytic enzymes; followed by contraction; fibroplasias; angiogenesis; and epidermal ingrowth.

Q: What is primary healing?
Ans: In surgical cases where the wound edges are opposed, healing proceeds rapidly to closure. This is known as primary healing.

Q: Why is healing by secondary intention a slower process?
Ans: Due to the formation and contraction of granulation tissue resulting in a slow apposition of the opposing skin appendages.

Q: What are complications of wound healing?
Ans: Incisional hernia, infection, inclusion cyst formation, pigmentation, hypertrophied scar, and contracture.

Q: Name the factors on which tensile strength of the healing wound depends.
Ans: On the amount and arrangement of the collagen fibres.

Q: Which local factors delay the process of healing?
Ans: Movement; infection; poor blood supply to wound; impairment of the lymph drainage; presence of foreign bodies; exposure to ionising radiation; exposure to ultraviolet light; type, size, and location of injury: necrosis; and amount of tissue separation in the wound.

Q: Deficiency of which nutrients delays the wound healing?
Ans: Deficiency of proteins (especially due to the deficiency of sulphur containing amino acids such as methionine), vitamin C (scurvy or malabsorption), vitamin A, and zinc.

Q: Which haematological abnormalities slow the process of wound healing?
Ans: Defect in neutrophil functions (chemotaxis and phagocytosis), neutropaenia, and bleeding disorders.

Q: Which cells can undergo hyperplasia?
Ans: 1. Labile cells (e.g. cells of the bone marrow and lymph nodes, epithelial cells of the skin and mucous membranes)
2. Stable cells (e.g. kidney, parenchymal cells of the liver, pancreas, adrenal, and thyroid gland) can undergo hyperplasia.

Q: Define metaplasia.

ONE-LINER QUESTIONS

Ans: Metaplasia is a pathological change, which refers to the reversible replacement of one type of differentiated cells with another type of mature differentiated cells.

Q: How dysplasia differs from metaplasia?
Ans: In dysplasia, normal differentiated cells are replaced by abnormal undifferentiated cells. In metaplasia, one type of differentiated epithelial cells is replaced by another type of normal differentiated epithelial cells.

Q: What are the types of necrosis based on aetiology and morphologic appearance?
Ans: Five types: coagulative, liquefaction (colliquative), caseous, fat, and fibrinoid necrosis.

Q: What is the characteristic of caseous necrosis?
Ans: It is characterised by the presence of cheese-like matter at the site of necrosis following infection with *Mycobacterium tuberculosis*.

Q: What series of sequential changes are likely to occur in the cell and its organelles as a result of apoptosis?
Ans: These include cell shrinkage (pyknosis), nuclear shrinkage, and condensation of chromatin, karyorrhexis, etc.

Q: Which are the most common cancers encountered in the developed countries and developing countries?
Ans: Developed countries: Lung, breast, prostate, and colorectal cancers
Developing countries: Liver, cervix, oral cavity, and oesophagus

Q: Group of conditions developing in patients with advanced cancer is known as?
Ans: Paraneoplastic syndromes

Q: Which is the specific marker for cancer of bowel, pancreas, and breast?
Ans: Carcinoembryonic antigen (CEA)

Q: Which is the specific marker for ovarian cancer and primary peritoneal cancer?
Ans: CA-125

Q: Which is the specific marker for breast cancer?
Ans: CA 15-3

Q: Which is the most frequently occurring arterial disease and is the commonest cause for arterial thrombosis?
Ans: Atherosclerosis

Q: Which is the major clinical syndromes resulting from ischaemia due to atherosclerosis in brain?
Ans: Transient cerebral ischaemia and cerebral infarcts or strokes

Q: How does the deep vein thrombosis develops?
Ans: Thrombophlebitis and infection of a lodged thrombus in a deep vein of the leg can result in the development of deep vein thrombosis

Q: Why is a pleural rub not a diagnostic feature for confirming the diagnosis of pulmonary embolism?
Ans: Because it may also be found on auscultation in cases of pneumonia.

Q: What are the classical findings on arterial blood gas analysis?
Ans: Hypoxia, hypocarbia, and increased alveolar-arterial oxygen gradient

Q: What is the treatment of pulmonary embolism?
Ans: Treatment requires systemic anticoagulation (heparin followed by warfarin)
In selected cases, such as central pulmonary embolism, surgical embolectomy may be performed.

Q: What are three stages of shock?
Ans: Initial reversible stage (compensated shock), progressive decompensated shock, and finally the stage of irreversible decompensated shock.

ONE-LINER QUESTIONS

Q: What is the mainstay of management for all forms of shock?
Ans: It is the maintenance of optimal tissue perfusion and ventilation through the administration of oxygen and intravenous fluids.

Q: Depending on the amount of blood loss, what are the types of haemorrhagic shock?
Ans: Compensated haemorrhagic shock (≤1,000 mL); mild haemorrhagic shock (1,000–1,500 mL); moderate haemorrhagic shock (1,500–2,000 mL); and severe haemorrhagic shock (>2,000 mL).

Q: What condition leads to the development of metabolic acidosis?
Ans: Tissue hypoxia

Q: Name the organisms causing septic shock.
Ans: Gram negative bacteria, e.g. *Escherichia coli, Aerobacter aerogenes, Bacillus proteus*, etc.
Gram-positive bacteria, e.g. diphtheria and gas gangrene.

Q: Which is the most common histological subtype of vulvar cancer?
Ans: Squamous cell cancer

Q: What are the main risk factors for developing vulvar cancer?
Ans: The presence of precancerous/dysplastic changes and chronic inflammation associated with lichen sclerosus, etc. in the vulvar tissues.

Q: Which is the type of epithelium lining the Fallopian tube?
Ans: Simple ciliated columnar epithelium

Q: What is the term used for the premalignant lesion in the vagina which can be described as a sequel to malignancy?
Ans: VAIN (vaginal intraepithelial neoplasia)

Q: Which investigation leads to diagnosis of cervical dysplasia/cervical intraepithelial neoplasia?

Ans: Cytological screening (Papanicolaou test or Pap smear) of the population

Q: Which is the most common type of carcinoma affecting the transformation zone?
Ans: Squamous cell carcinoma

Q: What are the risk factors for cervical cancer?
Ans: 1. Disorders of immune system (e.g. AIDS)
2. Young age at the time of first sexual intercourse
3. Having multiple sexual partners
4. History of smoking cigarettes

Q: Which is the most common gynaecologic cancer and known as the fourth most common cancer amongst women?
Ans: Endometrial cancer

Q: Which is the most common symptom associated with endometrial cancer?
Ans: Abnormal uterine bleeding

Q: What are the characteristics of adenomyosis?
Ans: Presence of nests or nodules of endometrium within the myometrial tissues (usually >2.5 mm beneath the basal endometrium).

Q: What is dysgerminoma?
Ans: It is another type of germ cell tumour of the ovary which is usually malignant in nature.

Q: What is threatened abortion?
Ans: The process of abortion has started, but has not progressed towards completion.

Q: In which abortion there is expulsion of products of conception en masse, following which there is subsistence of pain or bleeding?
Ans: Complete abortion

ONE-LINER QUESTIONS

Q: Which is the most common underlying cause for first and early second trimester miscarriages?
Ans: Chromosomal abnormalities

Q: Which chromosomal anomalies lead to first and early second trimester miscarriages?
Ans: Trisomy, polyploidy, monosomy, and structural chromosomal aberrations

Q: Which is the most common cause for late second-trimester spontaneous miscarriage?
Ans: Ascending infection of the genital tract with either localised inflammation in the region of cervical os or chorioamnionitis.

Q: Which immunological disorders are usually responsible for causing second trimester miscarriage?
Ans: Autoimmune and alloimmune including antiphospholipid syndrome

Q: What is characteristic feature of Mayer-Rokitansky-Kuster-Hauser syndrome (MRKH syndrome)?
Ans: There is an absence or hypoplasia of the internal vagina and absence of Fallopian tubes and uterus.

Q: How does MRKH syndrome occurs?
Ans: It occurs due to defect in fusion of the Mullerian ducts resulting in absence of proximal one third of vagina with or without the uterus.

Q: Which of the vulval skin disorders is associated with the highest risk of malignancy?
Ans: Lichen sclerosus

Q: What is the genotype in a case of complete molar pregnancy?
Ans: 46XX

Q: Which obstetric complication has an increased prevalence in women with bicornuate uterus?

Ans: Breech presentation

Q: Which cell is responsible for caseous necrosis in case of tuberculosis?
Ans: Macrophages

Q: What is the type of acute tubular necrosis of kidney?
Ans: Coagulative necrosis

Q: What is the most likely histological subtype of endometriosis associated with ovarian cancer?
Ans: Clear cell carcinoma

Q: Which type of necrosis is brain necrosis?
Ans: Colliquative necrosis

Q: What is the pathological mechanism occurring in breast tissue of a lady breastfeeding for 1 year?
Ans: Lobular hyperplasia

Q: What can be the increased risk for the lady who is suffering from lichen planus?
Ans: Squamous cell carcinoma

Q: In which subsites does vulvar cancer most commonly arise?
Ans: Labia majora

Q: Which human papillomaviruses (HPVs) is associated with an increased risk of cervical cancer?
Ans: HPV 16 and 18

Q: Which test is used to check ovarian reserves in pre-menopausal women?
Ans: Anti-Müllerian hormone

Q: What is the cause of thrombosis in protein C and S deficiency?
Ans: Antithrombin III

ONE-LINER QUESTIONS

CHAPTER 5
Microbiology

Q: Which of the following micro-organisms is responsible for causing chronic osteomyelitis after implant surgery?
Ans: *Staphylococcus aureus*

Q: Which of the following micro-organisms is responsible for causing pseudomembranous colitis?
Ans: *Clostridium difficile*

Q: Which microorganism cause suppurative urethritis in males?
Ans: *N. gonorrhoeae*

Q: Which of the following micro-organisms is responsible for causing gas gangrene?
Ans: *Clostridium perfringens*

Q: Strictly anaerobic bacteria are also known as:
Ans: Obligate anaerobes

Q: What are the examples of obligate anaerobes?
Ans: Clostridia, Bacteroides, and Actinomyces

Q: What are the examples of facultative anaerobic bacteria?
Ans: *Staphylococcus aureus, Escherichia coli, and* Listeria

Q: Which are the toxins and enzymes produced by *S. pyogenes?*
Ans: Toxins: Streptolysin O, streptolysin S, and pyrogenic exotoxins (erythrogenic, dick, and scarlatinal toxins).
Enzymes: Streptokinase (fibrinolysin), deoxyribonucleases (streptodornase DNase), hyaluronidase, proteinase, serum opacity factor, and nicotinamide adenine dinucleotidase (NADase).

Q: Which are the two post-streptococcal sequelae found in untreated infections?

Ans: Rheumatic fever following respiratory infection and glomerulonephritis following respiratory or skin infection

Q: Mention respiratory infections caused by Streptococcus?
Ans: Sore throat, streptococcal pharyngitis, scarlet fever, suppurative complications (e.g. peritonsillar or retropharyngeal abscess, otitis media, mastoiditis, quinsy, Ludwig's angina (diffuse cellulitis of the floor of the mouth), suppurative adenitis, etc.

Q: What are the main causes leading to acute glomerulonephritis in children in the tropics?
Ans: Impetigo (pyoderma) and streptococcal infection of scabies lesions

Q: Which is the most common cause of major neonatal infection?
Ans: Group B β-haemolytic Streptococcus (GBS)

Q: Which organism is responsible for majority of deaths due to maternal infection in the UK?
Ans: Group A streptococcus

Q: What are the latest recommendations by RCOG regarding the administration of intrapartum antibiotic therapy, if GBS is detected during the current pregnancy?
Ans: As per the latest guidelines by the RCOG (2017), first-line agent of choice in these cases is intravenous benzylpenicillin, which should be administered as soon as possible. If there is a history of a non-severe penicillin allergy then an injectable cephalosporin (eg cefuroxime) should be used. Intravenous vancomycin is recommended for women reporting a severe penicillin allergy.

Q: Which is the commonest aetiology for meningitis in the newborn babies?
Ans: Group B *Streptococci*, which may be acquired during or after delivery

Q: What is a frequent presentation of sepsis in the newborn?
Ans: Apnoeic episodes

ONE-LINER QUESTIONS

Q: Which bacteria has been recognised as an important cause of endocarditis and an important cause of nosocomial infection?
Ans: Vancomycin-resistant enterococci (VRE)

Q: What causes the inability to alter cell wall in VRE?
Ans: It is due to the fact that the vancomycin-sensitive precursor genes have been turned off and the resistant ones only appear in the presence of vancomycin.

Q: Which is the treatment of choice for Vancomycin-resistant enterococci?
Ans: High-dose ampicillin, only if the minimal inhibitory concentration of ampicillin is not too high

Q: Which test is used to distinguish S. aureus from coagulase-negative species?
Ans: The slide or tube coagulase

Q: Which are the two species of staphylococci?
Ans: 1. The coagulase-positive (e.g. S. aureus) and 2. coagulase-negative staphylococci (e.g. S. epidermidis and S. saprophyticus).

Q: What are the characteristics of the strains of S. aureus?
Ans: 1. It produces a golden-yellow colony pigmentation and haemolysis on blood agar.
2. Coagulase positive
3. Ferment mannite
4. Liquefy gelatin
5. Produce phosphatase
6. Black colonies on potassium tellurite blood
7. Produce thermostable nucleases which can be demonstrated by the ability of boiled cultures to degrade DNA in an agar diffusion test.

Q: Name the toxins produced by S. aureus.
Ans: 1. Five cytolytic or membrane-damaging toxins [alpha, beta, delta, gamma, and Panton-Valentine (P-V) leucocidin]
2. An enterotoxin, toxic shock syndrome toxin-1 (TSST-1)

3. Epidermolytic (exfoliative toxins)

Q: Which cutaneous infections are caused by Staphylococcus?
Ans: Furuncles or boils (large cutaneous abscesses), wound and burn infection, pustules (small cutaneous abscesses), carbuncles, styes, impetigo, and pemphigus neonatorum.

Q: Which deep infections are caused by Staphylococcus?
Ans: Endocarditis, osteomyelitis, periostitis, tonsillitis, renal abscess, pharyngitis, sinusitis, bronchopneumonia, empyema, septicaemia, meningitis, breast abscess, and abscesses in other organs.

Q: Who gets affected by toxic shock syndrome (TSS)?
Ans: TSS is a multisystem disease that primarily afflicts menstruating young women using tampons.

Q: What is SSSS? Name its causative organism.
Ans: It is an exfoliative skin disease in which the outer layer of epidermis gets separated from the underlying tissues. The epidermolytic toxin produced by *S. aureus* is responsible for the SSSS.

Q: Which was the first compound developed to combat resistance due to penicillinase (beta lactamase) production by staphylococci?
Ans: Methicillin

Q: Name the agents of choice in the treatment of systemic infection with MRSA.
Ans: Glycopeptides (vancomycin or teicoplanin)

Q: Which Mycobacteria causes skin ulcers?
Ans: *M. ulcerans* and *M. balnei*

Q: Which microorganism is known as Johne's bacillus?
Ans: *M. paratuberculosis*

Q: Name the saprophytic mycobacteria.
Ans: *M. butyricum*, *M. phlei*, and *M. stercoris*

ONE-LINER QUESTIONS

Q: What is the composition of Lowenstein-Jensen (LJ) medium?
Ans: It consists of coagulated hens' egg, mineral salt solution, asparagine and malachite green, glycerol, or sodium pyruvate.

Q: Which is the definite method to detect and identify *M. tuberculosis* and is sensitive and specific?
Ans: Culture examination

Q: What type of cells are clue cells?
Ans: Epithelial cells

Q: Which organism is a gut commensal, found in the intestinal tract of animals and humans and resists freezing?
Ans: Listeria monocytogenes

Q: What are the two types of listeriosis infection?
Ans: Non-invasive infection: Fall in the category of "flu-like illness". Complete recovery usually occurs in these cases.
Invasive: It is a serious generalised infection affecting the immunocompromised, the pregnant, and vulnerable groups like neonates and the elderly.

Q: Which diseases are caused by Listeria monocytogenes during pregnancy?
Ans: Miscarriage, stillbirth (up to 20% of cases), neonatal septicaemia, and neonatal death.

Q: If meconium is found in the liquor before 34 weeks, it could be associated with which possibility of foetal infection producing enteritis?
Ans: *Listeria monocytogenes*

Q: How is *Neisseria meningitidis* transmitted? What are the diseases caused by it?
Ans: Spreads via the droplet spread of respiratory secretions. It may be associated with bacteraemia and meningitis.

Q: How is bacteriological diagnosis of *Neisseria meningitidis* done?

Ans: It requires culturing of the cerebrospinal fluid obtained through lumbar puncture.

Q: Which is the most favourable medium for growth of Gonococci?
Ans: They grow well on chocolate agar and Thayer-Martin medium (chocolate agar containing vancomycin, colistin, and nystatin).

Q: Which is the primary site of infection in Gonococci infection in women?
Ans: Endocervix is the primary site of infection and extends to the urethra and vagina, giving rise to mucopurulent discharge.

Q: Which non-venereal infection is caused by Gonococci?
Ans: Ophthalmia neonatorum (amongst the newborn). This may be associated with a severe purulent eye discharge and periorbital oedema within a few days of birth.

Q: Which bacterium has highly pleomorphic structure with Chinese letter or cuneiform arrangement?
Ans: *Corynebacterium*

Q: What are Babes-Ernst granules?
Ans: The granules in the cell of *Corynebacterium* are known as metachromatic granules, volutin granules, or Babes-Ernst granules.

Q: Which are the two media useful for culturing *Corynebacterium*?
Ans: Löffler's serum slope and Tellurite blood agar

Q: Which test is used to distinguish susceptible individuals from those immune to diphtheria?
Ans: Schick's test. By injecting diphtheria toxins intradermally and observing for oedema and erythema (maximal in 2–4 days) in susceptible individuals.

Q: What are Diphtheroids?
Ans: These are bacteria belonging to the genus *Corynebacteria* resembling *C. diphtheriae* (occurring as normal commensals in the throat, skin, and other areas).

ONE-LINER QUESTIONS

Q: In which specie of Clostridium, spores may be subterminal or central?
Ans: *C. perfringens*

Q: What is Nagler reaction?
Ans: An opalescence in serum or egg-yolk media due to the production of phospholipase C.

Q: Which bacterium gives positive Nagler reaction?
Ans: *Clostridium perfringens*

Q: Which are the two distinct toxins produced by germination of tetanus spores?
Ans: An oxygen-labile haemolysin (tetanolysin) and a neurotoxin (tetanospasmin)

Q: Which organism is non-capsulated, motile with peritrichous flagella, and produces spores which are oval, subterminal, and bulging?
Ans: *Clostridium botulinum*

Q: Which are the three biovars (biological variants) of *Chlamydia trachomatis*?
Ans: Three biovars of *Chlamydia trachomatis* include: those which cause trachoma, those causing inclusion conjunctivitis (the so-called TRIC agents), and those causing lymphogranuloma venereum (LGV) and genital infections, respectively.

Q: Which are the two types of sexually transmitted genital tract infections caused by *C. trachomatis*?
Ans: 1. First one caused by the oculogenital serotypes D through K collectively referred to as "genital chlamydiasis".
2. The second type is LGV caused by serotypes L1, L2, and L3. LGV usually presents with swollen inguinal lymph nodes, which may have been preceded by one or more painless genital papules or ulcers.

Q: What is Reiter's syndrome?

Ans: Reiter's syndrome (found in men) is a triad of recurrent conjunctivitis, polyarthritis, and urethritis or cervicitis. It is associated with many infections but most commonly with *C. trachomatis*.

Q: What is the characteristic of Mycoplasma, which makes it unique amongst bacteria?
Ans: Absence of cell wall and a cell membrane containing sterols

Q: Mycoplasma was previously known as?
Ans: Pleuropneumonia like organisms or PPLO

Q: What is the appearance of Mycoplasma on agar colonies?
Ans: On agar, colonies are typically biphasic that have a "fried egg" appearance.

Q: Which Gram-negative enteric bacilli family is the largest, most diverse collection of medically important bacilli?
Ans: The Enterobacteriaceae family

Q: Name the genus of bacteria which are lactose fermenting and non-lactose fermenting.
Ans: Lactose fermenting: *Escherichia, Klebsiella,* and *Enterobacter*
Nonlactose fermenting: *Proteus, Shigella,* and *Salmonella*.

Q: Which is the most common agent associated with the UTI and gastroenteritis?
Ans: *E. coli*

Q: Which are the most common anaerobic bacteria in descending order?
Ans: *Bacteroides, Clostridia*, and *Peptostreptococci*.

Q: Which is the sensitive method for direct detection of treponemal antigens in the exudates for diagnosis of syphilis?
Ans: Direct fluorescent antibody test (DFA-TP)

Q: What is the incubation period of syphilis?
Ans: 9–90 days

ONE-LINER QUESTIONS

Q: What is hard chancre?
Ans: Primary lesion in syphilis is called chancre. It is circumscribed, painless, relatively avascular, indurated, superficially ulcerated lesion. It is covered by a thick, glairy exudate very rich in bacteria. This is known as "hard chancre".

Q: Which are the major types of serologic tests for syphilis?
Ans: Two types:
1. *Nontreponemal tests*: (Cardiolipin or lipoidal used as antigen) Flocculation tests, includes venereal diseases research laboratory (VDRL) test and rapid plasma reagin (RPR)
2. *Treponemal tests*: (Treponemes are used as the antigen) *T. pallidum* immobilization test (use live *T. pallidum* strains), *T. pallidum* agglutination test, *T. pallidum* immune adherence test, and fluorescent treponema antibody test (use killed *T. pallidum*), or *T. pallidum* hemagglutination test and enzyme immunoassay (use *T. pallidum* extracts as antigens).

Q: Which is the drug of choice for treating infections with *T. pallidum*?
Ans: Penicillin

Q: Which are the causative agent of relapsing fever, vincent's angina, and Lyme disease?
Ans: Relapsing fever: *B. recurrentis*
Vincent's angina: *B. vincentii*
Lyme disease: *B. burgdorferi*

Q: What are the three stages of Lyme disease?
Ans: *Stage 1*: (Incubation period of 3–30 days) "Localised infection" appears as a small red macule or papule at the site of bite (erythema migrans).
Stage 2: (Usually develops after weeks or months of the first stage) "Disseminated infection" develops with headache, fever, myalgia, and lymphadenopathy. Some develop meningeal or cardiac involvement.

Stage 3: (Sets in months or years later) "Persistent infection" appears with chronic arthritis, polyneuropathy, encephalopathy, and acrodermatitis.

Q: Which is the most common zoonotic bacterial disease throughout the world and name its causative organism?
Ans: Leptospirosis, caused by Leptospira

Q: What are the symptoms of leptospirosis?
Ans: 1. Mild virus-like syndrome (including symptoms such as fever, myalgia, headache, pneumonia, and jaundice)
2. Systemic leptospirosis with aseptic meningitis
3. Overwhelming disease (Weil's disease) with vascular collapse
4. Thrombocytopenia
5. Haemorrhage
6. Hepatic and renal dysfunction.

Q: Which microorganisms are traditionally considered to be transitional forms between bacteria and fungi?
Ans: Actinomycetes

Q: Name the five clinical forms of actinomycosis.
Ans: Cervicofacial, thoracic, abdominal, pelvic, and punch actinomycosis

Q: Which is the selective medium for *P. aeruginosa?*
Ans: Cetrimide agar

Q: Name the infections caused by *Pseudomonas aeruginosa*.
Ans: *Community acquired infections*: Corneal infections; otitis externa and varicose ulcers; industrial eye injuries; and contact lens-acquired infection.
Hospital-acquired infections: Infection in burns; localised lesions (infections of wounds and bedsores, eye infections, and urinary infections following catheterisation); skin lesions; iatrogenic meningitis; post-tracheostomy pulmonary infection; septicaemia, and endocarditis; infection of the nail bed; infantile diarrhoea and sepsis; osteomyelitis; infections of the gastrointestinal tract, CNS, and musculoskeletal system.

ONE-LINER QUESTIONS

Q: What is the source of transmission of Campylobacter in humans?
Ans: It is transmitted to humans by milk or water infected by wild and domestic animals and poultry.

Q: What is Hill's criteria?
Ans. Hill's criteria include a set of nine criteria, which help provide epidemiologic evidence of a causal relationship between a presumed cause and an observed effect. Hill suggested that there should be a dose-response relationship, that is, higher levels of the causative factor should lead to more severe disease or more rapid disease onset. Moreover, removing the factor of interest is likely to reduce the risk of disease.

Q: What are pathogenicity and virulence?
Ans: Pathogenicity is the ability of a microbial species to cause a disease.
Virulence is the ability of a strain of a species to produce disease.

Q: What are the most powerful human poisons known?
Ans: Bacterial protein toxins

Q: What are the sources of exogenous pyrogens and endogenous pyrogens?
Ans: *Exogenous pyrogens*: Infective agent, immunological reactions, or toxins
Endogenous pyrogens: Cytokines such as IL1 and IL6, tumour necrosis factors-β, and interferon-α.

Q: Name the factors which influence performance of a disinfectant.
Ans: 1. *pH of the medium:* Many organisms have an optimum pH at which they work best.
2. *Temperature*: Warm liquid disinfectants are more effective than colder ones.
3. *Numbers of organisms*: Higher number of organisms lead to clump formation.
4. *Concentration of disinfectant*: The concentration of disinfectant as well as the type of organisms is also important.

Q: Which is the method of choice for sterilisation of metal instruments (such as forceps, scissors, and scalpels)?
Ans: Hot air oven

Q: What is tyndallization?
Ans: An exposure of steam at 100°C for 20 minutes on three successive days is called tyndallization or intermittent sterilisation.

Q: Name the phenol derivatives commonly used as antiseptics.
Ans: Cresol, chlorhexidine, chloroxylenol, and hexachlorophane.

Q: Which dyes are used extensively as skin and wound antiseptic agents?
Ans: Aniline and acridine

Q: What are the most common types of hospital-acquired infections?
Ans: Bloodstream infections, pneumonia (ventilator-associated pneumonia), UTI, and surgical site infections

Q: What is the incubation period in infective-toxic type of food poisoning?
Ans: 6–12 hours

Q: Name the examples of toxic type of food poisoning.
Ans: Staphylococcal food poisoning, poisoning by *Bacillus cereus,* and *C. botulinum.*

Q: Which viruses are included in Herpesviridae family of viruses?
Ans: It consists of double-stranded (ds) DNA viruses that include herpes simplex, varicella zoster, cytomegalovirus (CMV), and Epstein-Barr virus (EBV).

Q: What is the unique property of herpesviruses?
Ans: These viruses are able to establish latent, lifelong persistent infections in their hosts, which can be periodically reactivated.

Q: Which virus can remain latent in the trigeminal ganglion and dorsal root ganglion and may reactivate as cold sores?

ONE-LINER QUESTIONS

Ans: Human herpesvirus 1

Q: Name the virus causing two distinct clinical entities in humans.
Ans: Varicella zoster virus (VZV) causes chickenpox (varicella) and herpes zoster or shingles, which are two distinct clinical entities in humans.

Q: Does genital herpes cause preterm delivery or spontaneous abortion?
Ans: No, genital herpes does not cause preterm delivery or spontaneous abortion.

Q: What is the mode of transmission of CMV?
Ans: CMV is transmitted orally and sexually, through tissue transplants, via blood transfusions, in utero, at birth, and by nursing.

Q: Which is the diagnostic feature of the cells infected by CMV?
Ans: Presence of "Owl's-eye" inclusion body and basophilic intranuclear inclusion body on histopathology

Q: Which is the most commonly available serologic test for measuring antibodies to CMV?
Ans: The enzyme-linked immunosorbent assay (or ELISA)

Q: What are the clinical features of congenital CMV infection?
Ans: Hepatosplenomegaly, microcephaly, sensorineural deafness, intracranial calcification, chorioretinitis, evidence of intrauterine growth restriction (IUGR), anaemia, jaundice, skin rashes, echogenic bowel, hearing loss, prolonged elevation of bilirubin, and rarely inguinal hernia.

Q: What is the mode of spreading of Varicella-zoster virus?
Ans: Respiratory and close contact

Q: How can CMV transmit from the mother to neonate?
Ans: The virus can be transmitted vertically from the mother: across the placenta, directly from the genital tract during delivery, and in breast milk.

Q: Name the tests used for diagnosis of Epstein-Barr virus.
Ans: Monospot test, ELISA, Western blot, DNA probe, PCR, and virus isolation

Q: What types of Human papillomavirus are "low-risk" and "high-risk"?
Ans: Types 6 and 11 are "low-risk" [associated with benign genital warts and low grades of cervical intraepithelial neoplasia (CIN)]. Types 16, 18, 30, 33 are "high-risk" [cause CIN lesions of all grades and cervical cancer, both squamous carcinoma (more common) and adenocarcinoma].

Q: Name two highly effective vaccines available in the UK for protection against HPV.
Ans: Cervarix and Gardasil. Cervarix protects against HPV types 16 and 18. Gardasil provides protection against types 16 and 18, and also immunises types 6 and 11.

Q: Which hepatitis virus is a DNA virus?
Ans: Hepatitis B virus (HBV) (belonging to the family Hepadnaviridae)

Q: What is the method of prevention of HAV?
Ans: By use of vaccines containing formalin-inactivated HAV. Prophylaxis with hepatitis A immunoglobulin can be administered to the contacts within 2 weeks of exposure.

Q: By what name is the Hepatitis B surface antigen also known as?
Ans: The Australia antigen

Q: Which molecular methods are used in diagnosis of HBV?
Ans: DNA hybridization and PCR

Q: Which drug is contraindicated in pregnancy in case of treatment of HCV infection?
Ans: Ribavirin

Q: Which are the specific diagnostic tests for infection due to HEV?

Ans: PCR to detect HEV RNA, and ELISA, which detects both IgG and IgM anti-HEV antibodies

Q: What are the characteristic features of Rubella?
Ans: This illness is characterised by mild exanthematous fever, transient macular rash (lasting for approximately 3 days), and lymphadenopathy.

Q: Which anomalies constitute the classical congenital rubella syndrome?
Ans: Patent ductus arteriosus, ventricular septal defects, sensorineural deafness, peripheral pulmonary artery stenosis, cataracts/congenital glaucoma, pigmentary retinopathy, purpura, splenomegaly, jaundice, microcephaly, mental retardation, meningoencephalitis, and radiolucent bone disease.

Q: Is rubella infection during pregnancy associated with a high risk of recurrent miscarriage?
Ans: Pregnancy during which primary rubella infection is contracted has a higher incidence of miscarriage. After that, rubella immunity is developed, which protects subsequent pregnancies from this complication.

Q: Which cells are principally infected by HIV virus?
Ans: CD4 lymphocytes

Q: What are the important structural components of the HIV?
Ans: The surface antigen gp120, the transmembrane antigen gp41, the matrix protein p17, and the capsid antigen p25.

Q: Define two types of serological tests for anti-HIV antibodies.
Ans: *Screening test*: includes ELISA
Supplementary tests: include the western blot and indirect immunofluorescence assay.

Q: What are the signs of toxicity due to the use of antiretroviral drugs?

Ans: Pre-eclampsia, liver dysfunction, lactic acidosis, glucose intolerance, diabetes, rashes, etc.

Q: Name the antiretroviral for which the most extensive safety data is available regarding use in pregnancy.
Ans: Zidovudine

Q: What combinations of drugs for the treatment of HIV should be avoided during pregnancy?
Ans: These include dual NRTI (non-reverse transcriptase inhibitors); combination of stavudine with didanosine (due to the risk of lactic acidosis), etc.

Q: Define types of infection caused by Candida.
Ans: *Superficial infection*: Mucocutaneous lesions (oral thrush, vulvovaginitis, balanitis, conjunctivitis, keratitis, etc.), and skin and nail infections.
Systemic infection: Intestinal candidiasis, bronchopulmonary candidiasis, septicaemia, endocarditis, meningitis, kidney infections, and UTIs.

Q: Which stain is used to identify *Toxoplasma gondii*?
Ans: Giemsa stain.

Q: What treatment protocol should be followed if foetus is infected with *Toxoplasma gondii*?
Ans: If the foetus is not infected, acute infection in pregnancy can be treated with spiramycin. In case the foetus is infected, a combination of sulphadiazine and pyrimethamine is used.

Q: What are the classic manifestations of vaginal trichomoniasis?
Ans: A purulent, frothy, yellow-greenish discharge with an abnormal odour, pruritus, and dysuria

Q: What is the shape of the protozoan *Trichomonas vaginalis*?
Ans: Pear-shaped

ONE-LINER QUESTIONS
CHAPTER 6
Immunology

Q: What is the main function of B-lymphocytes?
Ans: To synthesise antibodies after binding of antigen to specific epitopes

Q: What is the high HIV viral load and what does it indicate?
Ans: The high HIV viral load can vary from 5,000 copies/mL to 10,000 copies/mL. It indicates that HIV is reproducing and that the disease will likely progress faster than if the viral load is low.

Q: What is the low HIV viral load and what does it indicate?
Ans. The low HIV viral load is usually between 40 copies/mL and 500 copies/mL. It indicates that HIV is not actively reproducing and that the risk of disease progression is low.

Q: What is the drug of choice for treatment of falciparum malaria in pregnancy?
Ans. Treatment of choice for severe falciparum malaria is IV artesunate. IV quinine may be used if artesunate is not available. Uncomplicated *P. falciparum* (or mixed infections, such as *P. falciparum* and *P. vivax*) can be treated with drugs such as quinine and clindamycin.

Q: Why is the primaquine contraindicated during pregnancy with malaria?
Ans. Primaquine should not be administered to anyone with glucose-6-phosphate dehydrogenase deficiency because there can be a severe reaction with haemolytic anaemia. Primaquine is contraindicated in pregnancy, because the glucose-6-phosphate dehydrogenase status of the foetus would be unknown.

Q: Which is the most common cause for caseous necrosis on biopsy?
Ans: Acid-fast bacillus (tuberculosis infection)

Q: Which is the most common cause for gastroenteritis in children?
Ans. Rotavirus

Q: Systemic lupus erythematosus (SLE) is what kind of hypersensitivity reaction?
Ans: Type III hypersensitivity

Q: Which phagocytic antigen cell is present in the cervix?
Ans: T-lymphocyte

Q: What kind of vaccine should not be given to pregnant woman?
Ans: Live attenuated vaccine

Q: What is the screening test for haemolytic anaemia?
Ans. Coomb's test

Q: Which antigen presenting cells are present in cervix?
Ans. Langerhans cells

Q: Wound infection caused by which microorganism shows sulphur granules under microscopy?
Ans. *Actinomycosis israelii*

Q: What is the most likely organism for causing greenish white coloured vaginal discharge and erythematous appearance cervix?
Ans. *Trichomonas vaginalis*

Q: Which of the following is the primary opsonin in the complement system?
Ans: C3b

Q: Which is the main immunoglobulin in the gut that secretes saliva, milk, tears, and is important in mucosal immunity?
Ans. IgA

Q: Which cells secrete both heparin and histamine?
Ans: Mast cells

Q: What does the Kleihauer test determine?

ONE-LINER QUESTIONS

Ans: Foetomaternal haemorrhage

Q: Natural killer cells belong to which cell type?
Ans. Lymphocytes

Q: What is the most common type of nosocomial infection in hospitals?
Ans: Urinary tract infection

Q: What is the most common organism that causes sepsis during pregnancy?
Ans: Group A *Streptococci*

Q: Which is the commonest commensal organism that form common flora in vagina?
Ans: *Doderlein's lactobacillus*

Q: On what basis does the Lancefield grouping of *Streptococci* takes place?
Ans: Carbohydrate antigen on cell wall

Q: Which one of the following congenital infections is most characteristically associated with foetal hydrops?
Ans: Parvovirus B19

Q: Which class of immunoglobulin mainly activate the classical complement system?
Ans: IgM

Q: What cell type is the "clue cell"?
Ans: Vaginal squamous epithelial cell

Q: When does vertical transmission of HIV infection occur?
Ans: During labour and delivery

Q: Which immunoglobulin class has a pentameric structure and is unable to cross the placenta?
Ans: IgM

Q: What is the most common infective cause of newborn anaemia in UK?
Ans: Parvovirus B19

Q: Which immunoglobulin gives passive immunity to foetus?
Ans: Immunoglobulin G

Q|: Which cells are found at inflammation site?
Ans: Neutrophil

Q: What is the mode of action of pertussis vaccine?
Ans: Killed (inactivated) vaccine

Q: Where does the synthesis of complement protein occur?
Ans. Liver

Q: Which cell type predominates in a postoperative patient who presents with redness of the skin around the scar and nodule?
Ans. Macrophages

Q: What is the mechanism of action of Botulinum toxin?
Ans: It affects the cholinergic system by blocking the release ofacetylcholine at the pre-synaptic level.

Q: Which organism can be predicted if the culture of the lady with intrauterine contraceptive device (IUCD) shows sulphur granules?
Ans. *Actinomyces*

Q: Which organism can be suspected to cause infection in a lady who has a boyfriend, is presented with vaginal discharge and the culture shows the presence of Gram-negative cocci?
Ans: *Neisseria gonorrhoeae*

Q: What percent of untreated individuals move on to the third stage of syphilis?
Ans: 35%

ONE-LINER QUESTIONS

Q: Which microorganism is most likely to be associated with bladder catheterisation?
Ans: *Pseudomonas aeruginosa*

Q: Which antibody (immunoglobulin) class is involved in the allergic reactions?
Ans: IgE

Q: Which class of immunoglobulin is primarily secreted in breast milk and protects the infant's intestinal mucosa from infection?
Ans. IgA

Q: Which of the following fungi is most commonly found in catheter-related infection?
Ans: *Candida* spp.

Q: Which of the following cell types lyses cells that have been infected with viruses?
Ans: CD8+ T cells

Q: What is the basic principle of the Kleihauer Betke test?
Ans: Foetal haemoglobin is resistant to acid elution

Q: Which is the main immunoglobulin in mucosa?
Ans. IgA

Q: Which is the most important complement in opsonisation?
Ans. C3b

Q: What is the origin of macrophage?
Ans. Monocytes

Q: Condylomata lata is seen in which stage of syphilis?
Ans: Secondary syphilis

Q: Which bacteria cause toxic shock syndrome?
Ans: *Staphylococcus aureus*

Q: Define types of lymphoid organs based on their function.
Ans: *Primary (central)*: Sites where lymphocytes mature and become antigenically committed. These include thymus and bone marrow.
Secondary (peripheral): Capture antigens and provide sites where lymphocytes become activated by interaction with antigens. These include spleen and the lymph nodes.

Q: How does size of thymus vary after birth and throughout the life?
Ans: It rapidly becomes double in size after birth and stays the same in size throughout life.

Q: Define humoral immunity and cell-mediated immunity.
Ans: *Humoral immunity (antibody-mediated)*: It results from the activation of naive lymphocytes (primary response) or memory lymphocytes (secondary response).
Cell-mediated immunity (cell-mediated): It is the specific immune responses which involve functions mediated via T-lymphocytes. There is no involvement of antibodies in the cell-mediated immunity.

Q: What are the factors influencing the level of innate immunity?
Ans: Age, hormonal influences, gender, nutrition, and stress

Q: Define mechanisms of innate immunity.
Ans: Cellular factors in innate immunity (e.g. macrophages); mechanical barriers and surface secretions; presence of antibacterial substances in blood and tissues (e.g. complement system); microbial antagonisms; and inflammation, fever, acute phase proteins, etc.

Q: Define types of acquired immunity.
Ans: Two types: active immunity and passive immunity

Q: What is composition of vaccines?
Ans: Vaccines could be composed of any of the following: live, attenuated microorganisms; killed microorganisms; microbial extract; vaccine conjugates; and inactivated toxoids.

ONE-LINER QUESTIONS

Q: The passive transfer of immunity from mother to baby through the placenta is an example of which type of immunity?
Ans: Natural passive immunity

Q: What is the origin of leucocytes?
Ans: Leucocytes originate from pluripotent stem cells in the foetal liver and in the bone marrow from where they migrate to other body sites.

Q: Which blood cells are responsible for both non-specific and specific immunity in humans?
Ans: The white blood cells (leucocytes)

Q: What are the types of lymphocytes?
Ans: B cells, T cells, and natural killer (NK) cells

Q: Name the factors on the basis of which T cells can be classified.
Ans: On the basis of their surface markers, major histocompatibility complex (MHC) restriction, target cells, and function.

Q: Where does maturation of B-cells takes place?
Ans: Bone marrow, Payer's patches

Q: Define the term CD.
Ans: The term CD refers to the family of surface glycoprotein antigens that can be recognised by specific antibodies produced against them.

Q: By which cells CD3 is expressed?
Ans: Only by T cells

Q: By which cells CD68 is expressed?
Ans: Only by macrophages

Q: How does self-MHC class II restriction help in antigen recognition?
Ans: MHC class II restriction helps in stimulating and promoting the growth of T cells and macrophages. They also help B cells to make

antibodies in response to antigenic challenge and stimulate cell-mediated immunity.

Q: What are the two subsets of helper cells (on basis of different profiles of cytokines produced)?
Ans: Th1 and Th2

Q: Define suppressor T cells.
Ans: Also called Ts cells. These have CD8 surface marker and MHC class I restriction. They can suppress the response of B cells and the T cells.

Q: Which cells are involved in delayed hypersensitivity and cell-mediated immune response?
Ans: Delayed type-hypersensitivity T cells (Td cells)

Q: Which cells are also called CD8+ cells? What is their function?
Ans: Cytotoxic T cells (Tc cells). They can kill and lyse target cells carrying new or foreign antigens (including tumour, allograft, and virus infected cells).

Q: Name the cells providing memory and an amnestic immune response.
Ans: Memory cells (Tm)—both CD4 and CD8 cells

Q: Where are the genes of the MHC are located?
Ans: On the short arm of human chromosome 6

Q: What does the MHC in humans is known as?
Ans: Human leucocyte antigen (HLA) complex

Q: Mention the cases in which HLA typing or tissue typing is performed?
Ans: Anthropological studies; tissue transplantation; disputed paternity; and an association between HLA types and diseases.

Q: What do B lymphocytes require for their maturation?
Ans: Bone marrow cytokines and stromal cells

ONE-LINER QUESTIONS

Q: What enables B cells to be capable of binding to erythrocytes coated with antibody and complement, forming EAC rosettes?
Ans: Presence of a C3 receptor (CR2) on the B cell surface

Q: From where are the Natural killer (NK) cells derived?
Ans: Large granular lymphocytes

Q: Natural killer (NK) cells form part of which type of immunity?
Ans: The innate immune setup

Q: Which factors are released by natural killer cells?
Ans: Interferon gamma (IFN-γ), granulocyte-macrophage colony stimulating factor, and colony stimulating factor 1

Q: What is the size of blood macrophages and tissue macrophages?
Ans: Blood macrophages (monocytes): 12–15 μm
Tissue macrophages (histiocytes): 15–20 μm

Q: What is the name given to macrophages in the liver, lung, connective tissues, liver, kidney, brain, and bone?
Ans: Liver—Kupffer cells; Lungs—alveolar macrophages; connective tissues—histiocytes; kidney—mesangial cells; brain—microglial cells; and bone—osteoclasts.

Q: What enables phagocytosis to be enhanced in the presence of fresh serum (though possible in a saline medium)?
Ans: This is due to presence of substances called opsonins.

Q: Is process of opsonisation MHC-restricted or not?
Ans: It is not MHC-restricted.

Q: What is the morphological characteristic feature of microphages?
Ans: These are characterized by the presence of granules in their cytoplasm.

Q: Why are granulocytes also called polymorphonuclear leucocytes?
Ans: Because of the presence of irregular-shaped nuclei, they are named polymorphonuclear leucocytes.

Q: How many types of dendritic cells are present?
Ans: Four types: Langerhans cells, interstitial dendritic cells, myeloid cells, and lymphoid dendritic cells.

Q: What is the composition of mast cells?
Ans: They contain storage granules that contain lytic enzymes (e.g. tryptase) and inflammatory mediators, (e.g. histamine, heparin, serotonin, leucotrienes, platelet aggregating factor, leucocyte chemotactic factor, hyaluronidase, etc.).

Q: What triggers the release of inflammatory mediators by mast cells?
Ans: Release of inflammatory mediators occurs during mast cell degranulation. This can be triggered by events such as drugs, complement activation, tissue injury, and foreign antigenic material.

Q: When does anaphylactic reaction occurs?
Ans: It occurs when a previously sensitised individual is re-exposed to the antigen. It is an IgE-mediated immune response.

Q: Name the determinants of antigenicity.
Ans: Susceptibility to tissue enzymes, size, chemical nature, foreignness, antigenic specificity, species specificities, etc.

Q: What is composition of antigens?
Ans: Antigens are usually proteins or polypeptide molecules. Large carbohydrate molecules may also be antigenic.

Q: What are super antigens?
Ans: These are bacterial proteins which can interact with T cells and antigen-presenting cells (APCs) in nonspecific manner.

Q: Where does production of immunoglobulin occurs and what is its molecular weight?
Ans: *Average molecular weight*: 100 kDa
Site of production: Ribosomes of plasma cells

ONE-LINER QUESTIONS

Q: What prevents the foetus from forming antibodies to its own proteins?
Ans: Antibodies are not formed in the blood during early foetal life. Immunological tolerance prevents the foetus from forming antibodies to its own proteins.

Q: Why is the response to the second antigenic exposure is greater in comparison to the first exposure?
Ans: Because the immune system has been already sensitised by the first exposure

Q: How many polypeptide chains are present in antibody molecule?
Ans: Four polypeptide chains: two identical light chains and two identical heavy chains

Q: What connects light chains and identical heavy chains present in antibody molecule?
Ans: These are linked by disulphide bonds.

Q: How many fragments are present in an immunoglobulin molecule?
Ans: Two fragments: FAB (antigen binding fragment) and Fc (crystalline fragment)

Q: Mention the types of antigenic determinants on immunoglobulins.
Ans: (1) Isotypes; (2) allotypes and (3) idiotypes

Q: What is immunoglobulin fold?
Ans: There is a characteristic tertiary structure in each of the domains in the immunoglobulin molecule. This is called the immunoglobulin fold.

Q: Name the diseases associated with abnormalities in immunoglobulins.
Ans: Multiple myeloma, heavy chain disease C, cryoglobulinaemia, etc.

Q: In plasma, what is the concentration of IgA?

Ans: 200 mg/dL

Q: What are the two forms of IgA? In which forms both of them exist?
Ans: Serum IgA and secretory IgA. Serum IgA occurs in the monomeric form. Secretory IgA occurs in a dimeric form.

Q: Which is the rarest type of immunoglobulin?
Ans: Immunoglobulin E

Q: Which immunoglobulin is involved in type I hypersensitivity mechanism?
Ans: Immunoglobulin E

Q: Which is the largest immunoglobulin?
Ans: Immunoglobulin M

Q: Which is the main function of IgM?
Ans: Complement fixation

Q: What type of immunoglobulin is cryoglobulin?
Ans: Immunoglobulin M

Q: Which Immunoglobulin constitute maximum of all immunoglobulins in a healthy individual?
Ans: IgGs. Approximately 75% of all immunoglobulins

Q: Name the immunoglobulin which freely crosses the placental barrier.
Ans: IgG

Q: Which immunoglobulin provides immune protection for the newborn in the first few months of life?
Ans: IgG

Q: Name the diseases caused by deficiencies in C2 and C4 components of the complement pathway.
Ans: Paroxysmal nocturnal haemoglobinuria and hereditary angioedema

ONE-LINER QUESTIONS

Q: Define primary immunodeficiency. Which immune functions are affected by it?
Ans: It is a condition resulting from a genetic or developmental defect in the immune system. It may affect either adaptive or innate immune functions.

Q: Define secondary immunodeficiency. Name the factors causing it.
Ans: It is the loss of immune function, resulting from exposure to various agents. It can result from use of immunosuppressive agents, malnutrition, infections (such as AIDS), and malignancies.

Q: Which mechanisms are involved in induction of autoimmunity?
Ans: Inappropriate class II MHC expression on cells, release of sequestered antigens, molecular mimicry, and polyclonal B cell activation

Q: What are the characteristic features of APS?
Ans: Placental abruption, recurrent foetal loss, impaired foetal growth, severe growth restriction, and premature delivery

Q: Mention the manifestations of APS.
Ans: Deep vein thrombosis (DVT), renal vein thrombosis, Addison's disease, stroke, epilepsy, myocardial infarction, valvular lesions, transient ischaemic attacks (TIAs), leg ulcerations, pulmonary hypertension (due to thromboembolic disease), etc.

Q: Which autoimmune disorder is associated with systemic lupus erythematosus (SLE): primary APS or secondary APS?
Ans: Secondary APS

Q: Name the two main antibodies present in cases of APS.
Ans: ACA (anticardiolipin antibody) and LA (lupus anticoagulant)

Q: At what time should screening for LA and ACA be done in all patients with recurrent miscarriage?
Ans: In the first trimester

Q: What is the standard management in cases of APS?
Ans: It comprises of low dose aspirin and heparin. These reduce the incidence of late pregnancy complications.

Q: Name the symptoms associated with worsening lupus nephritis during pregnancy.
Ans: Proteinuria, oedema, thrombocytopenia, and raised blood pressure.

Q: What causes neonatal SLE?
Ans: It results from passively acquired maternal anti-Ro antibodies.

Q: What treatment is given to the mothers once the neonatal lupus is detected in the foetus?
Ans: High-dose corticosteroids and plasmapheresis

Q: Which diseases are associated with use of penicillamine during pregnancy?
Ans: Cutis laxa, inguinal hernia, and joint hypermobility

Q: Which complication is associated with use of azathioprine during pregnancy?
Ans: Intrauterine growth restriction

Q: Which are four different basic types of transplants?
Ans: Autograft, isograft, allograft, and xenograft

Q: What is allograft?
Ans: It is tissue transferred between genetically different members of the same species.

Q: Which is the strongest force in rejection in transplantation?
Ans: The immune response to tissue antigens encoded within the MHC is the strongest force in rejection in transplantation.

Q: Name the three important components which are required for graft-versus-host reaction to occur.
Ans: (1). The donor graft must contain immunocompetent T cells. (2). The host must be immunocompromised so that the graft cannot

be rejected. (3). The recipient should express antigens such as MHC proteins, which will be identified as foreign to the donor.

Q: Name the types of hypersensitivity reactions.
Ans: Types I, II, III, IV, and V

Q: Which type of hypersensitivity reaction is known as immediate hypersensitivity?
Ans: Type I hypersensitivity reaction

Q: What are the clinical manifestations of type I hypersensitivity reactions?
Ans: Generalised or systemic anaphylaxis or localised anaphylactic (type I) reactions

Q: Which type of reaction is seen in the cases of atopy and anaphylaxis following exposure to allergens, e.g. peanuts?
Ans: Type I hypersensitivity reaction

Q: What causes type II hypersensitivity reactions, or cytotoxic reactions?
Ans: Antibodies (IgG or IgM)

Q: Mention some type II hypersensitivity reactions.
Ans: Transfusion reactions, pernicious anaemia, Goodpasture's disease, and haemolytic disease of the newborn

Q: Which type of hypersensitivity reaction causes SLE?
Ans: SLE is caused by type III hypersensitivity.

Q: Which cells play an important role in type III hypersensitivity reaction|?
Ans: T-cells

Q: Name two types of delayed hypersensitivity reactions.
Ans: Tuberculin or Mantoux reaction and contact dermatitis

Q: Name the three pathways involved in complement cascade activation. What are the factors activating these pathways?
Ans: The classical, alternative, or mannose-lectin pathways.
Classical pathway: Activated with the formation of soluble antigen-antibody complexes (immune complexes) or the binding of antibody (IgG or IgM) to antigen on a suitable target, such as a bacterial cell.
Alternative pathway: Activated by the action of microbial polysaccharides and aggregated IgA or IgG.
Mannose lectin pathway: Activated by lectins.

Q: What is the central component between all the three pathways?
Ans: C3

Q: What is amplification loop?
Ans: C3Bb can become a C3 convertase, which amplifies the system, thus triggering more C3b formation. This is known as the amplification loop. It causes amplification of both classical and alternative pathways involved in the complement cascade.

Q: What is the composition of vaccine against *H. influenzae* (used in the UK)?
Ans: It is made from capsular polysaccharide (extracted from cultures of Hib bacteria). The polysaccharide is conjugated to a protein. Hib vaccines are conjugated with either CRM197 (a non-toxic variant of diphtheria toxin) or tetanus toxoid.

Q: What is mode of administration of Hib vaccine?
Ans: Deep subcutaneous or intramuscular injection

Q: In which combinations Hib vaccine is given?
Ans: It is given as part of a combined product: diphtheria/tetanus/acellular *pertussis*/inactivated polio vaccine/*Haemophilus influenzae* type b (DTaP/IPV/Hib) vaccine.

Q: What is the recommended age of children for DTaP/IPV/Hib?
Ans: From 2 months up to 10 years of age

Q: What is the recommended amount of DTaP/IPV/Hib for vaccination?

ONE-LINER QUESTIONS

Ans: The prescribed amount consists of three doses of a Hib-containing product with an interval of 1 month between each dose.

Q: What is the composition of MMR vaccine?
Ans: It is freeze-dried, and contains live attenuated measles, mumps, and rubella viruses.

Q: What is the composition of MMR 2 (Merck) vaccine?
Ans: It contains the Edmonston strain of measles, RA27/3 of rubella, and Jeryl Lynn strain of mumps.

Q: What is the site of administration of MMR vaccine?
Ans: It is administered intramuscularly into the upper arm or anterolateral aspect of thigh.

Q: What is the site of administration of MMR vaccine in patients with bleeding disorders?
Ans: Deep subcutaneous injections

Q: What are the absolute contraindications to MMR vaccinations?
Ans: Children with allergies to neomycin or kanamycin; a severe reaction to previous MMR; untreated cancer or diseases of the immune system; and children receiving immunosuppressive therapy or high dose steroids.

Q: What are the relative contraindications to MMR vaccinations?
Ans: An acute febrile illness; administration of another live vaccine within 3 weeks of proposed MMR vaccination; administration of immunoglobulins within 3 months of the proposed MMR vaccine; allergy to egg (in such case administration should be in a supervised, controlled environment); and should be avoided in pregnant women for 1 month (because of rubella).

Q: How levels of IgG and IgD vary in pregnancy?
Ans: IgG decreases in pregnancy.
IgD increases in pregnancy.

Q: Which test is used to quantify fetomaternal transfusion?

Ans: The Kleihauer Betke test

Q: Which test is used for detecting the maternal antibodies attached to the foetal cells?
Ans: The direct Coomb's test

Q: Why Direct Coomb's test is positive in cases where methyldopa has been administered?
Ans: Because methyldopa causes drug-induced, immune-mediated haemolysis

Q: Mention the cases in which Direct Coomb's test is positive.
Ans: 1. Cold antibody autoimmune haemolysis: Atypical pneumonia due to mycoplasma, infectious mononucleosis, paroxysmal cold haemoglobinuria, etc.
2. Haemolytic disease of the newborn
3. Warm antibody autoimmune haemolysis: SLE
4. Methyldopa has been administered
5. Usage of cephalosporins

ONE-LINER QUESTIONS
CHAPTER 7
Embryology

Q: Why does facial nerve of the baby get injured during vaginal delivery?
Ans: Mastoid process is underdeveloped

Q: Which structure develops into kidney and renal duct?
Ans: Metanephros

Q: In which phase of eukaryotic cell division, the cell can go into quiescent stage?
Ans: G0

Q: At which stage the DNA is checked?
Ans: G_2 checkpoint

Q: In the foetal circulation umbilical venous blood passes through which structure before entering the inferior vena cava passes?
Ans: Ductus venosus

Q: Through which structure blood passes from inferior vena cava to left ventricle in foetal circulation?
Ans: Foramen ovale

Q: What is the rule of primitive streak?
Ans: Migration of mesoderm

Q: At which gestational age there is maximum number of ova?
Ans: 20 weeks

Q: What is the likely gestation age when foetal poles are seen but heartbeat not visible?
Ans: 5 weeks

Q: Which drug may result in positive Coomb's test?
Ans: Methyldopa

Q: Where does the sperm penetrate at fertilization?
Ans: Zona pellucida

Q: Which hormone does corpus luteum produce?
Ans: Progesterone

Q: When is the heartbeat first seen on ultrasound?
Ans: Day 22

Q: At the end of which phase of the cell cycle the mutation of genes is controlled?
Ans. G1

Q: What organ removes old red blood cells?
Ans: Spleen

Q: Which of the following is homologous to the female paroophron and epoophron?
Ans: Paradidmyis (duct of epoophron resemble duct of epididymis)

Q: Which region of the placenta is in direct contact with maternal side?
Ans: Maternal endothelium

Q: From where is the new non-invasive prenatal diagnostic test of cell-free foetal DNA of maternal blood derived?
Ans: Foetal RBCs

Q: From what part of the embryo does primordial germ cell orginate?
Ans: Yolk sac endothelium

Q: Which cells are mainly responsible for producing premenopausal oestrogen?
Ans: Ovarian granulosa cells

Q: What is the embryological origin of bladder trigone?
Ans: Mesonephric duct

ONE-LINER QUESTIONS

Q: What is the embryological origin of allantois?
Ans: Endoderm

Q: What is embryological remnant of mesonephric duct?
Ans: Gartner's cyst

Q: Through which shunt does blood passes from umbilical vein into inferior vena cava (IVC)?
Ans: Ductus venosus

Q: The structure produced after the first meiotic division?
Ans: Primary oocyte

Q: In which stage of the cell cycle does mitosis proceeds?
Ans: M Phase

Q: What is the name of structure that shunts oxygenated blood from the right to left atrium in the foetus?
Ans: Foramen ovale

Q: Primitive gonads develop from which cell layer?
Ans: Intermediate mesoderm

Q: Which is the immediate layer around the oocyte of the tertiary follicle?
Ans: Zona pellucida

Q: The ureteric bud is derived from which of the following embryonic structures?
Ans: Mesonephric duct

Q: The vertebral column is developed from which germ layer?
Ans: Paraxial mesoderm

Q: The two medial umbilical folds represent remnants of which structure?
Ans: Obliterated umbilical arteries

Q: Which of the following is in direct contact with maternal blood in lacunae of the placenta?
Ans: Chorion

Q: Inhibin is secreted by which cell type of the ovary?
Ans: Granulosa cells

Q: Which types of cells are phagocytic for residual bodies left over from the process of spermiogenesis?
Ans: Sertoli cells

Q: Chromosomes arrange themselves on equatorial plate in which phase of the cell cycle?
Ans: Metaphase

Q: How many telomeres are present in the cell during metaphase of mitosis?
Ans: 4

Q: Which remnant of mesonephric duct is seen during laparoscopy?
Ans: Epoöphoron

Q: What is the correct relation of round ligament with its embryological origin and anatomy?
Ans: Mesoderm and in front of uterine cornu

Q: Which layer surrounds the zona pellucida?
Ans: Cumulus oophorus

Q: The lower part of vagina is derived from which part?
Ans: Endoderm

Q: What is the embryological origin of Gartner duct?
Ans: Mesonephric duct

Q: What is the embryological origin of gonadotrophin-releasing hormone (GnRH)?
Ans: Hypothalamus

ONE-LINER QUESTIONS

Q: What is gastrulation?
Ans: Formation of the primitive streak and the intra-embryonic mesoderm

Q: In which phase replication of chromosomes occurs?
Ans: In the S phase

Q: Which structure acts as the coordinating centre for the cells microtubules?
Ans: Centrosome

Q: What causes anaphase lag to occur?
Ans: Delayed movement of chromatids during mitosis or one homologous chromosome during meiosis can cause anaphase lag.

Q: What causes trisomy or development of cells with 47 chromosomes?
Ans: As a result of anaphase lag, an extra chromosome can get incorporated into the nucleus of the other daughter cell, which is characterized by the presence of an extra chromosome in the normal diploid.

Q: What causes production of isochromosomes?
Ans: Division of the chromatids in an abnormal plane results in production of isochromosomes

Q: Which one is reductional division: Meiosis I or Meiosis II?
Ans: Meiosis I is a reductional division. Meiosis II is an equational division.

Q: When does meiosis begins in males?
Ans: At the time of puberty during spermatogenesis

Q: When does meiosis begins in females?
Ans: Meiosis in the ovaries begins before birth even though it is actually completed just prior to ovulation.

Q: When do primordial germ cells reach the developing gonads?
Ans: These cells start migrating towards the developing gonads by 4th week, where they reach by the end of 5th week.

Q: Where do primordial germ cells originate?
Ans: These originate in the wall of the yolk sac.

Q: Which hormones control the process of spermatogenesis?
Ans: Follicle-stimulating hormone and testosterone

Q: What is the role of FSH in the regulation of spermatogenesis?
Ans: It stimulates the production of testicular fluid.

Q: What is the role of LH in the regulation of spermatogenesis?
Ans: It helps in the regulation of spermatogenesis and influences production of testosterone.

Q: Which cells are equivalent to the granulosa cells of the ovary?
Ans: Sertoli cells

Q: Where are the male germ cells present at the time of birth?
Ans: In the sex cords of the testis in the form of large pale cells surrounded by supporting cells, also known as the Sertoli cells

Q: What is the time required for the completion of the entire process of development of spermatozoon from the spermatogonium?
Ans: About 70–75 days

Q: What is normal sperm count?
Ans: 10^8/mL

Q: When does the development of testes occur in the genital ridge?
Ans: After 7 weeks of gestation

Q: When does peak synthesis of testosterone occurs in the period of gestation?
Ans: Between 15 to 18 weeks of gestation. After that there is a decline in its synthesis.

ONE-LINER QUESTIONS

Q: Which cells secrete testosterone in males and females?
Ans: Males—interstitial cells of Leydig in testes
Females—adrenal cortex in females

Q: Where does fertilization takes place?
Ans: In the ampulla of the uterine tube

Q: How much time does fertilized egg take to travel to the implantation site?
Ans: 5 to 7 days

Q: When does implantation of blastocyst occurs?
Ans: About 6–7 days after fertilisation

Q: What is the most common site of implantation?
Ans: Upper posterior wall of the uterine cavity

Q: At which stage chromosomes start occupying the equatorial plane of the mitotic spindle?
Ans: Metaphase

Q: How many rounds of DNA replication occurs during two successive phases of meiosis?
Ans: Only one round

Q: How many chromosomes are present in secondary spermatocytes?
Ans: 23 chromosomes

Q: How many spermatids are produced from each diploid spermatocyte?
Ans: Four spermatids

Q: Which hormone induces the development of male secondary sexual characteristics?
Ans: Male androgen (testosterone)

Q: From where are the Müllerian ducts derived?

Ans: Coelomic epithelium

Q: What is the embryological origin of paramesonephric ducts?
Ans: They develop from coelomic epithelium on the urogenital ridge.

Q: What is the embryological origin of interstitial cells of Leydig?
Ans: Mesenchyme

Q: Which structures arise from the Wolffian ducts?
Ans: Epoöphoron, paroöphoron, Skene's gland, and Gartner's duct

Q: What is the embryological origin of Fallopian tubes?
Ans: Müllerian ducts

Q: What results in formation of double uterus?
Ans: It may result from failure of fusion of the Müllerian ducts.

Q: Up to what gestational age mesonephric and paramesonephric ducts coexist in all embryos?
Ans: Up to 8 weeks of gestation

Q: What determines the development of the testes?
Ans: It is determined by the presence of SRY gene.

Q: When does urine formation begins in foetal life?
Ans: Urine formation begins at about the 3rd month of foetal life, and continues increasing volume till term.

Q: How much amount of urine is voided by mature foetus into the amniotic cavity?
Ans: 450 mL

Q: What is the embryological origin of urinary bladder?
Ans: It is derived in part from the urogenital sinus, and in part from the ends of the mesonephric ducts.

Q: When does foetal heart starts contracting?
Ans: At 3 weeks gestation

ONE-LINER QUESTIONS

Q: At what time does placental circulation starts?
Ans: It starts at about 1 week after implantation.

Q: When does heart becomes a four-chamber organ?
Ans: At about 7 weeks' gestational age

Q: At what gestational stage embryo is called foetus?
Ans: When the embryo becomes 7 or 8 weeks old, it is known as a "foetus".

Q: Which structure decides the axis of the embryo, which can now be divided in two lateral halves, the right and the left?
Ans: The prochordal plate

Q: Which structure is at the cephalic end of the embryo?
Ans: The oral membrane is at the cephalic end of the embryo and is the future mouth.

Q: Which organ has dual origin (developing both from the foetus and the mother)?
Ans: The placenta

Q: Which structure attaches the maternal and foetal component of placenta to one another?
Ans: Cytotrophoblastic shell

Q: What is "after birth"?
Ans: During parturition, the decidua is shed off along with the placenta and membranes (amnion and chorion) which are sometimes also known as the "after birth".

Q: When does development of the chorionic villi takes place?
Ans: Around 12th day after fertilisation, development of the chorionic villi takes place.

Q: Which structure functions to transfer oxygen and other important nutrients between mother and foetus?
Ans: Chorionic villi

Q: What is weight of placenta?
Ans: About 500 grams

Q: How many blood vessels are present in mature umbilical cord?
Ans: Three large blood vessels: two umbilical arteries (bringing foetal blood to the placenta), and a single umbilical vein (returning blood to the baby's heart).

Q: Mention the layers of placental membrane starting from the maternal side.
Ans: 1. Syncytiotrophoblast; 2. cells of cytotrophoblast; 3. basement membrane of cytotrophoblast; 4. mesoderm; and 5. endothelium and basement membrane of the branches of umbilical blood vessels (foetal blood) in the villi.

Q: Which hormones are synthesized by placenta?
Ans: Progestins and oestrogens, hCG, relaxin, and human placental lactogen

Q: What is primitive streak?
Ans: A linear raised area formed over the superior surface of the embryonic disc towards the caudal end of the embryo due to linear proliferation of the ectodermal cells along the central axis of the embryo near the tail.

Q: What is the embryological origin of mammary gland?
Ans: Ectoderm

Q: Name the factors which determine the phenotypic sex.
Ans: It is determined by the appearance of external genitalia and secondary sexual characteristics (which develop at the time of puberty).

Q: What comprises the urogenital ridge?
Ans: Mesonephros and genital ridge

Q: Which structure connects the primitive kidney (Wolffian body or mesonephros) to the cloaca?

ONE-LINER QUESTIONS

Ans: The Wolffian duct

Q: Which structure helps in storing the sperms?
Ans: Vas deferens

Q: Mention the embryological remnants of the mesonephric tubules in the males.
Ans: The paradidymis; the ductulus aberrans inferior; and the ductulus aberrans superior

Q: When do the Leydig cells of foetal testis begin to secrete testosterone?
Ans: At 8–9 weeks of gestation

Q: What is the effect of abnormal androgen exposure between 9th to 14th week of gestation in males and females?
Ans: *Males*: External genitalia does not undergo complete masculinization. This results in development of a small phallus, hypospadias, and scrotal defects.
Females: This results in varying degree of masculinisation such as clitoral hypertrophy and labial fusion.

Q: What is the embryological origin of vagina?
Ans: Vagina is derived from sinovaginal bulbs and from the vaginal plate.

Q: Which developmental stage of kidney is responsible for the formation of the majority of the urogenital system in humans and is functional well before birth?
Ans: The metanephros

Q: What is the embryological origin of Bowman's capsule and the glomerulus?
Ans: Metanephros

Q: At what gestational age the kidneys attain their adult position?
Ans: During the 8th week of foetal life

Q: What is the embryological origin of the trigone of the bladder and the posterior wall of the urethra?
Ans: Mesonephric ducts

Q: Which pharyngeal arch is an abortive arch that disappears soon after its formation and no trace of its nervous or vascular elements are left?
Ans: The 5th arch

Q: Name the pre-trematic nerve of first arch.
Ans: Chorda tympani

Q: Muscles of pharynx, soft palate, and cricothyroid are derived from which pharyngeal arch?
Ans: Fourth arch

Q: What is value of foetal haemoglobin concentration?
Ans: Between 17 to 19 g/dL

ONE-LINER QUESTIONS
CHAPTER 8
Genetics

Q: which test helps in the diagnosis of Cystic fibrosis?
Ans: Sweat test

Q: What hormone is deficient in congenital adrenal hyperplasia?
Ans: 21-Hydroxylase deficiency

Q: What is the genetic composition of Klinefelter syndrome?
Ans: 47,XXY

Q: How is cystic fibrosis detected?
Ans: Chorionic villus sampling (CVS) and amniocentesis

Q: What is the second common enzymatic deficiency after 21-OH in CAH?
Ans: 11-beta hydroxylase

Q: How many genes encoded in mitochondrial DNA?
Ans: 37 genes

Q: What is the name of the chromosome rearrangement that involves the transfer of genetic material between two non-homologous chromosomes?
Ans: Robertsonian translocation

Q: What role does messenger RNA play in the synthesis of proteins?
Ans: Transcription

Q: How does Robertsonian translocation occur?
Ans: Breaks at or near the centromeres of two acrocentric chromosomes followed by the reciprocal exchange of broken parts

Q: What is the smallest human chromosome?
Ans: Chromosome Y

Q: An inherited metabolic disorder called phenylketonuria (PKU) can result in serious problems in infancy. Describe the inheritance pattern of PKU.
Ans: Autosomal recessive

Q: What is the mode of inheritance of Duchenne muscular dystrophy (DMD)?
Ans: X-linked recessive

Q: Which of the following is the genotype of Edward's syndrome?
Ans: 47,XX

Q: Which structure is predominantly affected by Sheehan's syndrome?
Ans: Anterior pituitary

Q: Which chromosome have centromere located at one side?
Ans: Submetacentric chromosome

Q: What is the chromosomal pattern of Turner's syndrome?
Ans: 45,XO

Q: What role does messenger RNA play in the synthesis of proteins?
Ans: Translation

Q: 46 XX karyotype is associated with which of the condition?
Ans: Constitutional hirsutism

Q: 46 XY karyotype is associated with which of the condition?
Ans: Testicular feminisation syndrome

Q: How many hydrogen bonds are present in guanine-cytosine bonds?
Ans: Three hydrogen bonds

Q: In which syndrome there are 11 pair of ribs?
Ans: Edward's syndrome

ONE-LINER QUESTIONS

Q: Which syndrome is associated with tall stature due to delayed fusion of the epiphysis?
Ans: Klinefelter's syndrome

Q: Which syndrome is characterised by the presence of colobomas in the iris?
Ans: Patau's syndrome

Q: Which syndrome occurs due to the abnormality of the testosterone receptors?
Ans: Testicular feminisation syndrome

Q: What is the most basic structural unit of DNA?
Ans: Nucleotide

Q: Describe the structure of nucleotide.
Ans: Each nucleotide subunit comprises of a phosphate, deoxyribose sugar, and one of the four nitrogenous bases.

Q: Mention nitrogenous bases in DNA and RNA.
Ans: *DNA*: Thymine, adenine, guanine, and cytosine (T, A, G, and C)
RNA: Uracil, adenine, guanine, and cytosine (U, A, G, and C)

Q: How many hydrogen bonds are present between adenine and thymine?
Ans: Two hydrogen bonds

Q: Which enzymes can separate hydrogen bonds between the strands of the double helix?
Ans: Helicases

Q: Mention the atmospheric conditions under which the two strands of the DNA helix denature and separate.
Ans: When heated to about 94° C for 5 minutes

Q: Which sequences are included in stop codons?
Ans: Sequences UAA, UGA, and UAG

Q: Name the disorders associated with the abnormality of trinucleotide repeats sequences.
Ans: Fragile X syndrome, Huntington's chorea, and myotonic dystrophy

Q: Mention the regulatory elements of gene transcription.
Ans: *Promoters*: regions of DNA to which RNA polymerase bind and initiate transcription
Enhancer sequences: modify activity of genes on the same chromosome
Transacting proteins: modify genes on both pairs of homologous chromosomes

Q: Define the process of translation.
Ans: It is a process in which the information in the mRNA is used to direct the synthesis of polypeptides on the ribosomes.

Q: Which organelle is only inherited from the mother and not inherited from the father?
Ans: The mitochondrial DNA

Q: Name the genetic conditions associated with mutations in the structure of mitochondrial DNA.
Ans: Leber's hereditary optic neuropathy, cytochrome C oxidase deficiency, Kearns-Sayre syndrome, Leigh syndrome, maternally inherited diabetes, deafness, etc.

Q: How many chromatid arms are present in a chromosome?
Ans: It consists of two identical chromatids which are held together in the midline at the centromere.
Short arm: Called as p (after the word "petit" meaning "small")
Longer arm: Called as q (as it is the next alphabet in the series after "p").

Q: Which test is used to distinguish between chromosomes that are similar in size and shape?
Ans: Q-banding

ONE-LINER QUESTIONS

Q: What term can be given to the occurrence of more than one morphological form in the population?
Ans: Polymorphism

Q: In which chromosomes length of both the arms is equal?
Ans: Metacentric chromosomes

Q: In which chromosomes the centromere is slightly away from the center?
Ans: Submetacentric chromosomes

Q: In which chromosomes chromosomal arm on one side is very long and that on the other side is very short?
Ans: Acrocentric chromosomes

Q: Which chromosomes are the acrocentric chromosomes seen in humans?
Ans: Chromosome numbers 13, 14, 15, 21, and 22

Q: Name the translocation in which the two chromosomes fuse at the centromere, giving rise to a translocation.
Ans: Robertsonian translocations

Q: Which chromosomes are not present in human cells?
Ans: Telocentric chromosomes (centromere is located at the terminal end of the chromosome)

Q: Which type of splitting of replicating chromosomes occurs in isochrome chromosomes?
Ans: In such chromosomes, transverse splitting of replicating chromosomes occurs. Because of this, two chromosomes having both identical arms are formed.

Q: How many Barr bodies are present in normal female somatic cells and normal male somatic cells?
Ans: Normal female somatic cells: One Barr body
Normal male somatic cells: No Barr body

Q: How many Barr bodies are present in females with XXX karyotype?
Ans: Two Barr bodies

Q: To which cells Lyon's hypothesis is not applicable?
Ans: Germ cells

Q: At what gestational age process of inactivation of X chromosome occurs?
Ans: Probably by day 16

Q: In how many cells of buccal smear from a woman can Barr body be seen?
Ans: In up to 30% of cells

Q: Presence of which extra chromosome is usually associated with mental retardation.
Ans: Presence of an extra X chromosome is usually associated with mental retardation.

Q: Which chromosome demonstrates fluorescence with quinacrine?
Ans: Y chromosome

Q: Which inheritance pattern is associated with presence of hairy ears?
Ans: Presence of hairy ears is associated with Y-linked inheritance pattern.

Q: What is the genetic composition of Hydatidiform mole?
Ans: 46,XX

Q: What is the genetic composition of Down syndrome?
Ans: Either 47,XX or 47,XY

Q: What is the genetic composition of polycystic ovarian syndrome?
Ans: 46,XX

Q: Which type of inheritance pattern is shown by Christmas disease and colour blindness?

ONE-LINER QUESTIONS

Ans: X-linked inheritance pattern

Q: Which pattern of inheritance is shown by neurofibromatosis?
Ans: Autosomal dominant inheritance pattern

Q: Which blood group is universal donor?
Ans: Blood group O

Q: Which blood group is universal recipient?
Ans: Blood group AB

Q: Which are the most common and rarest blood groups in the United Kingdom?
Ans: *Most common*: Blood group O
Rarest: Blood group AB

Q: Which pattern of inheritance is shown by Hurler's syndrome?
Ans: Autosomal recessive mode of inheritance

Q: Name the conditions in which polygenic or multifactorial inheritance occurs.
Ans: Diabetes mellitus; rheumatoid arthritis; neural tube defects (NTDs); and cardiac defects

Q: Which genetic disorders are associated with genetic anticipation?
Ans: Huntington's disease, myotonic dystrophy, and fragile X syndrome

Q: Define aneuploidy.
Ans: Aneuploidies can be defined as karyotypic disorders having an abnormal number of chromosomes (both autosomes and sex chromosomes).

Q: Which is the most commonly encountered trisomy?
Ans: Trisomy 16

Q: Cri du chat syndrome is associated with deletion of which chromosome?

Ans: It is associated with a deletion on the short arm of fifth chromosome.

Q: What results in Philadelphia chromosome?
Ans: It is the result of a reciprocal translocation between chromosome 9 and 22.

Q: Which is the most common type of congenital heart diseases present in Down syndrome?
Ans: Atrial septal defect

Q: Which test is used as screening test for Down syndrome?
Ans: Nuchal translucency

Q: Which blood parameters are measured in Triple test?
Ans: Alpha-fetoproteins, human chorionic gonadotropins, and unconjugated oestriol levels

Q: Which blood parameters are measured in Quadruple test other than the parameters measured in Triple test?
Ans: Inhibin A

Q: Edward's syndrome is characterised by the presence of three copies of chromosome ....
Ans: 18

Q: Clenched hand with the index finger overlapping the middle finger or middle finger overlapping the ring finger is associated with which syndrome?
Ans: Edward's syndrome

Q: Patau's syndrome is due to trisomy of which chromosome?
Ans: Chromosome 13

Q: Single palmer crease is associated with which syndrome?
Ans: Patau's

Q: Which genetic abnormality is associated with hypogonadism, infertility, and/or azoospermia in males?

ONE-LINER QUESTIONS

Ans: Klinefelter's syndrome

Q: By which techniques sperm retrieval can be done in most men with Klinefelter's syndrome?
Ans: MESA (micro-epididymal sperm aspiration) or TESE (testicular sperm extraction)

Q: What causes testicular feminisation syndrome?
Ans: It results due to the abnormality of the testosterone receptors.

Q: Which pattern of inheritance is shown by androgen insensitivity syndrome?
Ans: X-linked pattern of inheritance

Q: What is the probable diagnosis in an individual with primary amenorrhoea and no apparent vagina?
Ans: Müllerian agenesis (Mayer-Rokitansky-Küster Hauser Syndrome)

Q: What results in Müllerian agenesis?
Ans: This syndrome occurs due to defect in fusion of the Mullerian ducts resulting in absence of proximal one-third of vagina with or without the uterus.

Q: What is the treatment of Müllerian agenesis?
Ans: 1. Creating an artificial vagina through the use of Frank's dilators
2. Surgical procedure (McIndoe's vaginoplasty) at the time the patient plans to get married

Q: What is the characteristic feature of 5-α Reductase Deficiency (5-ARD)?
Ans: Virilization of the affected individuals to varying degrees at the time of puberty

Q: Which is the most common cardiac anomaly associated with Turner's syndrome?
Ans: Aortic valve disease

Q: What is the main manifestation of Triple X syndrome?
Ans: Woman affected with syndrome may have IQ lower than that of her siblings on the IQ scale by 10 points or more.

Q: Deficiency of which factor cause Haemophilia A and haemophilia B?
Ans: *Haemophilia A*: Deficiency of factor VIII
Haemophilia B: Deficiency of factor IX

Q: In whom haemophilia more likely to occur: males or females?
Ans: Males

Q: At what age patients suffering from haemophilia present with bleeding due to minor trauma?
Ans: In the first year of their life

Q: Which factor's deficiency causes Von Willebrand's Disease? What are its characteristic features?
Ans: Deficiency of vWF (Von Willebrand factor). This disease is characterised by abnormalities in coagulation and a variety of bleeding tendencies such as menorrhagia, easy bruising, bleeding from gums or nose, etc.

Q: Which is the most commonly observed symptom of Duchenne muscular dystrophy?
Ans: The weakness of the proximal muscles of the leg and pelvis along with the loss of muscle mass

Q: Which symptoms are associated with clinical triad of McCune-Albright syndrome?
Ans: Precocious puberty; Café au lait spots; and polyostotic fibrous dysplasia of bones

Q: Which disease has become the most common cause of significant neonatal jaundice worldwide (occurring within the first 3 days of life)?
Ans: Glucose-6-phosphate-dehydrogenase (G6PD) deficiency

ONE-LINER QUESTIONS

Q: Name the chemicals which can trigger G6PD deficiency.
Ans: Anti-malarial drugs such as primaquine, chloroquine and quinine; antibiotics like quinolones, e.g. nalidixic acid, and ciprofloxacin; mothballs containing naphthalene; and consumption of Fava bean.

Q: Which disease is known as Favism?
Ans: Favism can be defined as haemolytic response to the consumption of fava beans.

Q: Mention types of α-thalassaemia.
Ans: Four types:
1. Four α gene deletions: Hb Bart's hydrops fetalis
2. Three α gene deletions: HbH disease
3. Two α gene deletions: α thalassaemia trait
4. One α gene deletion: α thalassaemia trait (carrier)

Q. What is the probability of having cystic fibrosis in a child whose one parent is normal and other parent is the carrier of the disease?
Ans: 0%

Q: What is the main defect in β thalassaemia?
Ans: It is that the defect of β globin chains results in the accumulation of excessive α chains within the RBCs.

Q: How are β thalassaemia and thalassaemia major detected?
Ans: Beta thalassaemia trait: Usually asymptomatic and is identified during the routine blood evaluations.
Thalassaemia major: Detected during the first few months of life, when the patient's level of foetal haemoglobin decreases.

Q: What are clinical features of β-thalassaemia?
Ans: 1. Appearance of anaemia in the first 4–6 months of life
2. Hepatosplenomegaly, extramedullary haematopoesis, and iron overload
3. Typical thalassaemic facies and malocclusion of jaws due to expansion of maxillary bones, resulting in "chipmunk" face

4. Cardiac failure and arrhythmias due to severe anaemia and iron overload
5. Skull may show hair-on-end appearance
6. Impaired immunity

Q: What are the findings of blood film in case of thalassaemia?
Ans: 1. Blood film showing severe microcytic hypochromic red cell morphology, marked anisopoikilocytosis, basophilic stippling, nucleated red cells, presence of tear drop, and target cells
2. Low MCV and an elevated reticulocyte count is a feature of thalassaemia.

Q: What is the treatment of thalassaemia?
Ans: *Thalassaemia minor*: Patients do not require any treatment.
Thalassaemia major: The aim is to maintain the haemoglobin level between 9–10 gm/dL through regular blood transfusions.

Q: Which disease is considered as the commonest hereditary disease in Caucasians?
Ans: Cystic fibrosis

Q: What is the mode of inheritance of cystic fibrosis?
Ans: Autosomal recessive

Q: Which test (performed 3 days after fertilization) helps in the detection of abnormal cystic fibrosis genes?
Ans: Pre-implantation genetic diagnosis

Q: Mutation of which gene causes cystic fibrosis?
Ans: CFTR (Cystic fibrosis transmembrane conductance regulator) gene

Q: What is the prognosis of pulmonary hypertension in a pregnant patient with cystic fibrosis?
Ans: Development of pulmonary hypertension in a pregnant patient with cystic fibrosis can prove fatal.

Q: Which population is most commonly affected by Tay-Sachs disease?

ONE-LINER QUESTIONS

Ans: Ashkenazi Jews

Q: Who is more affected by fragile X syndrome: males or females?
Ans: Males. Despite of being a dominant condition, women are not usually affected because in women only one X chromosome remains active, which is usually the normal one (Lyon's Hypothesis).

Q: State True or False: Regular national screening program for fragile X syndrome exists in the UK.
Ans: False. (Regular national screening program for this disease exists in Australia, but not in the UK.)

Q: Which syndrome is considered as the most common inherited cause of mental retardation and the second commonest genetic cause of mental retardation (first being the Down syndrome)?
Ans: Fragile X syndrome

Q: Which syndrome is considered as the most common known cause of autism?
Ans: Fragile X syndrome

Q: What is associated with Fragile X syndrome: large ears or low set ears?
Ans: Large ears

Q: A 27-year-old female developed insulin dependent diabetes mellitus. Her uncle and grandmother also had diabetes mellitus. What is the most likely mode of inheritance for her condition?
Ans: Polygenic

Q: What are the causes of ambiguous genitalia at birth?
Ans: Congenital adrenal hyperplasia; maternal ingestion of androgenic or potentially androgenic drugs; maternal masculinising tumour; inadequate masculinisation of male foetus; and true hermaphroditism.

Q: Which is the most common cause of ambiguous genitalia?
Ans: Congenital adrenal hyperplasia

Q: What is the chromosomal pattern in hermaphroditism?
Ans: 46,XX

Q: What are the level of luteinising hormone/follicle-stimulating hormone ratio (LH/FSH) in patients with gonadal dysgenesis?
Ans: Level of luteinising hormone/follicle-stimulating hormone ratio is elevated.

Q: Mitochondrial genes are inherited from the mother/father?
Ans: Mother

ONE-LINER QUESTIONS
CHAPTER 9
Biophysics

Q: What is the frequency of transvaginal USG?
Ans: 7.5 MHz

Q: What is the frequency of transabdominal ultrasonography?
Ans: 3.5 MHz

Q: What is the frequency of current used in electrosurgery?
Ans: 100 KHz to 4Mhz

Q: Which of the following potential mechanism is more likely to cause tissue damage from ultrasound exposure?
Ans: Cavitation

Q: The standard chest X-ray is equivalent to what duration of natural background radiation?
Ans: 2–10 days

Q: On which basis ionising radiation can be categorized in to different types?
Ans: On the basis of the nature of the particles or the electromagnetic waves which create the ionising effect

Q: Which particle is identical to helium particles?
Ans: Alpha particle

Q: How many protons and neutrons are present in alpha particle?
Ans: Two protons and two neutrons

Q: What are the properties of beta particle?
Ans: It is a negatively charged particle known as electron. It has high speed and high energy.

Q: Which substances emit beta particles?
Ans: Radioactive nuclei

Q: Which particles are commonly used for PET scanning?
Ans: Positrons

Q: Which ionising radiations are electromagnetic radiations?
Ans: Gamma rays

Q: How are gamma rays produced?
Ans: They are produced during the process of γ-decay from the naturally occurring radioisotopes and are generated from the nucleus.

Q: Which ionising radiations are electromagnetic radiations generated by the circulating electrons?
Ans: X-rays

Q: What is the term given to thickness of a material, which will reduce their ionization to half its initial value as a measure of the penetrating power of the X-rays or gamma rays?
Ans: Half value layer

Q: What is considered as the most dominant marker of the activity of radiation?
Ans: Ionisation

Q: Which processes are likely to produce new chemical species within the cell?
Ans: Excitation and ionisation

Q: Which processes are imperfect ionizations in which the energy is imparted to the outer electrons of the atom to put them into orbits of energy higher than their usual?
Ans: Excitations

Q: Which is the most important mode of cell destruction by ionizing radiations?
Ans: DNA disruption

Q: What is the SI unit for the measurement of radioactivity?

ONE-LINER QUESTIONS

Ans: Becquerel (Bq)

Q: Define one Becquerel.
Ans: It is defined as one transformation (or decay or disintegration) per second.
1 Bq = 1 transformation per second

Q: Define "half-life".
Ans: The time required for half the initial quantity of radioactive material to complete its transformation.

Q: Name the diseases which can be associated with children exposed in utero to X-ray irradiation.
Ans: Childhood leukaemias and cancers (e.g. acute lymphoblastic leukaemia, cerebral gliomas)

Q: Mention sources of radiation in clinical practice.
Ans: *Ionising radiation*: X-ray; radiotherapy; positron emission tomography; barium studies (e.g. barium swallow, meal, enema, etc.); and CT scan.
Non-ionising radiation: Electrocautery; laser; MRI; ultrasound; microwaves; and diathermy

Q: What is the frequency of ultrasound waves?
Ans: Between 16–16,000 cycles per second

Q: What is piezoelectric effect?
Ans: Ultrasound waves are generated by the effect of electricity on a ceramic crystal. This is known as the piezoelectric effect.

Q: What frequency is used in medical ultrasound?
Ans: Between 1 million and 10 million cycles per second

Q: Which ultrasound is used to determine the velocity of blood flow?
Ans: Doppler ultrasound

Q: Name various types of Doppler ultrasounds which can be used to determine the velocity of blood flow.

Ans: Pulsed waves, continuous, and colour ultrasound

Q: Mention two principal bio-effects of ultrasound.
Ans: *Thermal*: This effect is created through the impact of acoustic energy upon tissue.
Mechanical: This bio-effect includes cavitation and streaming associated with the violent agitation of particles within the medium.

Q: When is anomaly scanning performed in pregnancy?
Ans: In the second trimester of pregnancy (conducted around 20 weeks of gestational age)

Q: At what gestational age foetal heart activity is usually visualized using transabdominal sonography?
Ans: At 6–7 weeks of gestation

Q: At what measurement of CRL absence of foetal heart activity implies non-viable pregnancy?
Ans: CRL of ≥7 mm

Q: Why vaginal transducers provide better resolution than abdominal transducers?
Ans: Vaginal transducers can use higher frequencies than abdominal transducers, thereby providing better resolution.

Q: Why sound waves weakens as they pass through the tissues?
Ans: Because parts of sound waves are reflected, scattered, absorbed, refracted, or diffracted.

Q: What is the unit of intensity?
Ans: Watts per centimetre square (W/cm^2)

Q: How is impedance related to the tissue density in case of soft tissues?
Ans: Impedance is proportional to the tissue density.

Q: What is the unit of impedance?
Ans: Impedance is measured in $g/cm^2/sec$.

ONE-LINER QUESTIONS

Q: How does ultrasound velocity varies with type of medium?
Ans: Ultrasound velocity in any given medium is constant.

Q: What is the main concern related with the use of ultrasound?
Ans: Main concern is the occurrence of thermal effects due to the heating of the local tissues.

Q: What are the acute side effects of radiotherapy?
Ans: Epithelial surface damage (e.g. mouth ulcerations); gastrointestinal damage (resulting in symptoms such as nausea, vomiting, abdominal pain); cystitis; fatigue; and oedema

Q: What are the late side effects of radiotherapy?
Ans: Lymphoedema; hair loss; further development of cancers; tissue fibrosis; and infertility

Q: What thermal index should be applied when using the transvaginal ultrasound during early pregnancy?
Ans: Thermal index must be preferably less than 1.

Q: How is Doppler shift related to the velocity of the reflector?
Ans: The Doppler shift is proportional to the velocity of the reflector.

Q: What is the principle of MRI?
Ans: Application of directional magnetic field, which causes change in the motion of the field of charged particles, forms the basis of MRI.

Q: Which process implies the use of electricity to generate heat in the tissues?
Ans: Diathermy/electrosurgery

Q: What is the use of diathermy at the time of surgery?
Ans: It is used to vapourise the tissues for cutting purposes or for coagulating the tissues to achieve haemostasis or for destroying the tissues.

Q: Which device is used to pass an electric current through tissues which causes coagulation, cutting, and tissue destruction by a heating effect?
Ans: Diathermy (or Bovie)

Q: What is the frequency of alternating current in process of diathermy?
Ans: 500 KHz–1 MHz

Q: What is the wave pattern of cutting diathermy and coagulation diathermy?
Ans: *Cutting diathermy*: Alternating sine-wave pattern
Coagulation diathermy: Damped or pulsed sine wave pattern

Q: What is the main advantage of use of high frequency in diathermy?
Ans: It is too fast to stimulate nerve fibres. This prevents spasm or paralysis of muscles.

Q: Which are the two types of diathermy commonly used in gynaecological surgery?
Ans: Unipolar and bipolar

Q: What are the uses of monopolar diathermy and bipolar diathermy?
Ans: *Monopolar diathermy*: Used to achieve cutting; to desiccate the tissues
Bipolar diathermy: Cutting is not possible with it; to desiccate the tissues

Q: Which type of diathermy is used at the time of using forceps? Why?
Ans: Bipolar diathermy. The current only flows between the tips of the forceps, from the active electrode to the neutral electrode. So there is a reduced risk of stray currents damaging tissues other that those, which are being aimed at.

Q: Which type of diathermy is used in laparoscopic surgery for dividing adhesions and myomectomy?

ONE-LINER QUESTIONS

Ans: Bipolar diathermy

Q: What are the uses of unipolar diathermy?
Ans: It used in surgery, including open, minimally invasive, colposcopic, and hysteroscopic.

Q: Why use of diathermy on the colon is an explosive risk?
Ans: Because colon contains hydrogen and methane.

Q: What should be the medium used to distend the abdomen at laparoscopy: combustible or noncombustible?
Ans: Noncombustible

Q: Why should non-conductive medium be used if diathermy is employed at the time of hysteroscopy?
Ans: Such medium is used so that the electric current does not get dissipated.

Q: Why should saline medium not be used if diathermy is employed at the time of hysteroscopy?
Ans: Saline is conductive. So, it is avoided.

Q: In which process the risks of thermal injury are minimal: unipolar diathermy or bipolar diathermy? Why?
Ans: Bipolar diathermy. Because the current only flows between the tips of the instrument, so heat is generated only at the tips. There is a small risk of damage from heated tissue coming into contact with other tissues.

Q: What is direct coupling?
Ans: A major complication associated with unipolar diathermy. It refers to the tissue damage caused by the electrode touching another nearby conducting instrument.

Q: What is expanded form of LASER?
Ans: LASER is an acronym for Light Amplification of Simulated Emission of Radiation.

Q: Which type of radiation is produced by LASER?
Ans: A laser produces a highly directional beam of coherent (monochromatic) electromagnetic radiation.

Q: Which is the most commonly used laser in medical practice?
Ans: Nd:YAG lasers (neodymium-doped yttrium aluminium garnet)

Q: What is the use of Nd:YAG laser?
Ans: It is commonly used for ablation of foetal vessels in cases of twin-twin transfusion syndrome.

Q: Which lasers are suitable for operating through thicker tissues and why?
Ans: Nd:YAG laser. Because its wavelength is in the near infrared range.

Q: What are the uses of carbon dioxide lasers?
Ans: These are also used for performing cone excisions from the cervix and for laser ablation of cervix.

Q: How many classes of lasers are present? Define them.
Ans: Four classes: Class 1; Class 2; Class 3 (divided into 3a and 3b); and Class 4

Q: To which class medical lasers belong?
Ans: Class 4

Q: What is the acoustic impedance?
Ans: The acoustic impedance of a material is the product of its density and the velocity of sound within it.

Q: What is velocity of ultrasound through the soft tissue?
Ans: About 1540 m/s

Q: Which classes of lasers are considered to be of low risk?
Ans: Class 1; Class 2; and Class 3a

Q: At what crown-rump length would it be expected to observe the foetal heart beat using transvaginal sonography?

ONE-LINER QUESTIONS

Ans: Greater than 2 mm

Q: Which type of diathermy necessitates the use of a return electrode?
Ans: Monopolar diathermy

Q: The standard chest X-ray is equivalent to what duration of natural background radiation?
Ans: 7–10 days

Q: A neutron has almost the same mass as a?
Ans: Proton

Q: A positron has the same size as an?
Ans: Electron

Q: What is the charge of a proton?
Ans: Positive

ONE-LINER QUESTIONS
CHAPTER 10
Epidemiology and Biostatistics

Q: What are the steps taken to promote, preserve and restore health in primary prevention of disease?
Ans: 1. Promotion of health-enhancing behaviours
2. Preventing the onset of at-risk behaviour

Q: What steps are involved in primary prevention in case of cervical cancer?
Ans: It involves reduction of smoking and promiscuous behaviour.

Q: What are the steps taken to promote, preserve, and restore health in secondary prevention of disease?
Ans: 1. Screening for risk factors and early detection of asymptomatic or mild cases
2. Starting an effective intervention and curative treatment

Q: What steps are involved in secondary prevention in case of cervical cancer?
Ans: Screening for detecting high risk cervical lesions which may be at a risk of becoming cancerous. Methods for screening of cervical cancer include cytological methods such as the traditional pap smear and thin layer preparation or the molecular biology methods such as HPV-DNA genotyping.

Q: What are the steps taken to promote, preserve, and restore health in tertiary prevention of disease?
Ans: 1. Helps in reduction of long-term impairment and disabilities
2. Helps in prevention of repeated episodes of clinical illness
3. Helps in slowing down the disease progression

Q: What steps are involved in tertiary prevention in case of cervical cancer?
Ans: Tertiary prevention in case of cervical cancer involves regular follow-ups of high grade and cancerous lesions.

Q: How does primary and secondary preventions effect disease epidemiology?
Ans: Primary prevention: Helps reduce the disease incidence
Secondary prevention: Helps reduce the disease prevalence

Q: What is point prevalence?
Ans: It is the proportion of all individuals with existing disease at a point in time.

Q: What is period prevalence?
Ans: The proportion of individuals with existing disease during a period of time.

Q: How is prevalence rate calculated?
Ans: Prevalence rate = $\dfrac{\text{Persons with existing disease at a given place at a given time}}{\text{Population of persons at risk for disease at a given place, at a given time}}$

Prevalence = Incidence × duration
Duration = Prevalence/Incidence

Q: What is "Number needed to treat"? How is it calculated?
Ans: NNT refers to number of individuals in general population, which need to be treated to prevent one case. It is the inverse of incidence. So if incidence is 20/1000, NNT = 50.

Q: Which indices are required for evaluating a clinical diagnostic test?
Ans: A clinical diagnostic test can normally be evaluated using four indices: sensitivity, specificity, positive predictive value, and the negative predictive value.

Q: Define "maternity".
Ans: Any pregnancy going to 24 weeks or beyond or one resulting in a live birth before 24 weeks.

Q: Define MMR as per WHO and UK.

ONE-LINER QUESTIONS

Ans: WHO definition of MMR: Number of "direct" and "indirect" deaths per 100,000 "live births".
UK definition of MMR: Number of 'direct' plus "indirect" deaths per 100,000 "maternities".

Q: Define indirect deaths.
Ans: Indirect deaths are deaths resulting from a previous existing disease, or disease that developed during pregnancy and which was not due to direct obstetric causes, but which was aggravated by the physiologic effects of pregnancy, e.g. cardiac disease.

Q: Define late maternal deaths.
Ans: Late maternal deaths can be defined as the deaths occurring between 42 days and 1 year after abortion, miscarriage, or delivery that are due to direct or indirect maternal causes.

Q: By which national programme are all maternal deaths in the UK and Ireland investigated?
Ans: All maternal deaths in the UK and Ireland are investigated by the national programme, the CEMD (confidential enquiries into the maternal deaths). These enquiries have been conducted in the UK since 1952. Since June 2012, the CEMD has been carried out by the MBBRACE-UK (Mothers and babies: reducing risk through audits and confidential enquiries).

Q: Name the countries where MBRRACE-UK system applies to?
Ans: The new MBRRACE-UK system applies to England, Wales, and Scotland.

Q: What was the topic for 2016 Confidential Enquiry into Maternal Morbidity (CEMM)?
Ans: Pregnancy in women with artificial heart valves

Q: What were the figures for the MMR for the years 2010–12 and 2012–14?
Ans: The figures for the MMR for the years 2010–12 and 2012–14 were 10 per 100,000 women and 8.5 per 100,000 women, respectively

Q: What are the most common cause of indirect maternal death and direct maternal death, according to MBRRACE UK (2016)?
Ans: *Indirect maternal death*: Cardiovascular disease (23% cases)
Direct maternal death: Thrombosis and thromboembolism (11% cases)

Q: What was the important cause of maternal mortality in the years 2011 and 2013?
Ans: Failure of recognition of signs of mental health disease

Q: What does 2014, 2015, and 2016 MBRRACE reports focused on?
Ans: *The 2014 MBRRACE report*: Maternal deaths and morbidity due to sepsis
The 2015 MBRRACE report: Maternal deaths due to psychiatric causes
The 2016 MBRRACE report: Maternal deaths due to cardiovascular diseases

Q: Which is the largest single indirect cause of maternal death during pregnancy and up to 6 weeks after pregnancy?
Ans: Cardiovascular disease

Q: Which is the leading cause of direct maternal death?
Ans: Thrombosis and thromboembolism

Q: How is perinatal mortality (PMR) defined?
Ans: PMR is defined as the number of stillbirths and deaths in the first week of life per 1,000 total deliveries.

Q: In UK, how is PMR calculated?

Ans:
$$PMR = \frac{\text{Total mortalities}}{\text{Total mortalities} + \text{Live births}} \times 1{,}000$$

Q: What is WHO criterion for PMR?

Ans: PMR for WHO ranges from stillbirths at 22 weeks (or babies born dead who are weighing >500 g in case the period of gestation is not known) to neonates less than 7 days of age

Q: What is UK criterion for PMR?
Ans: The legal definition of a stillbirth in UK is a baby delivered at or after 24 completed weeks of gestation showing no signs of life, irrespective of the time of death

Q: Which organization calculates PMR in UK?
Ans: In the UK, PMR is calculated on an annual basis by the Confidential Enquiry into Stillbirths and Deaths in Infancy (CESDI), set up in 1992.

Q: How does PMR varies with age in women?
Ans: PMR is lowest in mothers belonging to the age group 25–29 years. It is higher amongst teenagers and women of advanced age (>35 years).

Q: What are the risk factors for increased PMR?
Ans: These include obesity, extremes of birth weight, poor maternal health, nulliparity, race (highest risk in non-hispanic women), smoking, and low levels of maternal education.

Q: Define neonatal death and early neonatal death.
Ans: *Neonatal death*: Deaths (per 1,000 live births) occurring within 28 days of birth.
Early neonatal deaths: Deaths occurring within 7 days of birth (first week of life).

Q: How is infant mortality rate defined?
Ans: Infant mortality rate (IMR) can be defined as number of infant death (deaths during first year of life) per 1,000 live births

Q: What are the features of Perinatal Mortality Surveillance Report by MBRRACE-UK (2016)?

Ans: PMR was approximately 6 per 1,000 births. Most important causes of neonatal deaths were complications occurring during the neonatal period, followed by the congenital anomalies. Preterm birth is another important cause of neonatal deaths, which can be reduced by maternal administration of corticosteroids prior to the delivery.

Q: Name the studies used for displaying the relationship between the exposure to a particular causative agent and the disease (in epidemiology).
Ans: Observational studies: Nature is allowed to take its course; no intervention is done.
Experimental studies: There is an intervention and the results of the study assess the effects of the intervention.

Q: What is case report?
Ans: It is an objective report of a clinical characteristic or outcome from a single clinical subject or event, n = 1. With case reports, there is no control group.

Q: What is case series report?
Ans: Case series report is an objective report of a clinical characteristic or outcome from a group of clinical subjects, n >1. No control group.

Q: What is cross-sectional study?
Ans: In these cases, the presence or absence of disease and other variables are determined in each member of the study population or in a representative sample at a particular time. The co-occurrence of a variable and the disease can be examined.

Q: What is a case-control study?
Ans: It is a study which identifies a group of people with the disease and compares them with a suitable comparison group without the disease. It is almost always retrospective.

Q: What are features of cohort studies or longitudinal studies?
Ans: 1. It involves the follow-up of individuals.
2. Subjects are recruited into cohort studies and followed-up over time to assess the incidence of a particular disease.

3. In case of a disease that has already been diagnosed, disease progression can be assessed.

Q: Why cohort studies are more important than the cross-sectional studies?
Ans: Because they provide more information on the incidence of events. These studies also allow temporal assessments to be made regarding whether the exposure preceded the outcomes of interest or not.

Q: How is data analysis done in cross-sectional study?
Ans: Chi-square to assess association

Q: How is data analysis done in case-control study?
Ans: Odds ratio to estimate risk

Q: How is data analysis done in cohort studies?
Ans: Relative risk and/or attributable risk

Q: What is attributable risk/absolute risk reduction?
Ans: It is defined as comparative probability asking, "How many more cases in one group?" AR can be defined as the incidence rate of the exposed group minus the incidence rate of the unexposed group.

Q: What are control group and an intervention group in a research trial?
Ans: *Control group*: It includes subjects who do not receive the intervention under study. The control group is used as a source of comparison to be certain that the experiment group is being affected by the intervention and not by other factors. In clinical trials, the control group is most often a placebo group. Note that control group subjects must be as similar as possible to intervention group subjects.
Intervention group: It includes the subjects which receive the intervention.

Q: What are the phases of a clinical trial?

Ans: 1. Pre-clinical phase: This phase comprises of laboratory/animal studies.
   2. Clinical phase: This phase comprises of 3 to 4 phases and during this phase, the therapy is administered to the human subjects.
   - *Phase 1*: Testing safety in healthy volunteers
   - *Phase 2*: Testing protocol and dose levels in small group of patient volunteers
   - *Phase 3*: Testing efficacy and occurrence of side effects in larger group of patient volunteers (several hundred to several thousand)
   - *Phase 4*: Also, known as the post-marketing surveillance studies, are sometimes conducted after regulatory appraisal. They are critical for updating the ongoing use of the therapy.

Q: Define recall bias.
Ans: Subjects fail to accurately recall events in the past. This is a likely problem in retrospective studies.

Q: What is late-look bias?
Ans: Individuals with severe disease are less likely to be reported in a survey because they might have died.

Q: What is confounding bias?
Ans: The factor being examined may be related to other factors of less interest. Unanticipated factors may make a relationship ambiguous or make it seem as if a relationship is present when there is no relationship in reality. More than one explanation can be found for the presented results. For example, a study comparing the relationship between exercise and heart disease in two populations when one population is younger and the other is older. There occurs confounding bias in this case because it is difficult to decide whether the differences in heart disease are due to exercise or to age.

Q: Define "dispersion". How it can be measured?

ONE-LINER QUESTIONS

Ans: It refers to the spread of data. Statistical dispersion can be measured with the help of parameters such as range, variance, and standard deviation.

Q: Define range.
Ans: Range denotes the total collection of values between the largest and the smallest observation. This indicates how widely varied the data is. It is calculated by subtracting the lowest value from the highest value.

Q Define variance
Ans: Variance can be defined as the spread of the observations. This is an indication of variability of the observations. To calculate the variance, each observation is subtracted from the mean, squared, added-up and divided by the number of observations minus one.

Q: what is standard deviation?
Ans: Standard deviation provides a good indication of distribution about the mean. The standard deviation is a summary of how widely dispersed the values are around the center. It is equal to the positive square root of the variance.

Q: Define a confidence interval (CI).
Ans: It is a statistical range with a specified probability that a given parameter lies within the range. A confidence interval specifies how far above or below a sample-based value the population value lies within a given range, i.e. from a possible high to a possible low. The true mean, therefore, is most likely to be somewhere within the specified range.

Q: Define Type I error (α error).
Ans: Type I error is the incorrect rejection of a null hypothesis when it is really true. This is also known as a false positive finding. This error asserts that the drug works when it really does not.

Q: Define Type II error (β error).
Ans: Type II error is failing to reject the null hypothesis when it is really false. This is also known as a false negative finding. This error

asserts that the drug does not work when it really does. β error = 1− Power

Q: What are ways to categorize different types of variables in statistics?
Ans: There are four ways: nominal, ordinal, interval and ratio scales.
1. Nominal: Used for labeling variables, without any quantitative value, e.g. gender (male or female); hair colour (black, brown, or white), control group versus the drug group, etc.
2. Ordinal: Measures non-numeric concepts (e.g. pain sensation)
3. Interval: Scale graded in equal increments (e.g. measurement of temperature in celsius scale, time and gestational age)
4. Ratio scales: It orders things and contains equal intervals, but it also has a true zero point (e.g. height and weight).

Q: Define "Forest Plot Chart".
Ans: It is a graphical representation of a meta-analysis. Commonly presented with two columns:
- The left-hand column lists the names of the studies in chronological order from the top downwards
- The right-hand column is a plot of the measure of effect (e.g. an odds ratio) for each of these studies (often represented by a square) incorporating confidence intervals represented by horizontal lines.

Q: What is Box-and-Whisker Plot?
Ans: It is graphical depiction of the groups of numerical data through their quartiles

Q: What is correlation?
Ans: This is the relationship between the two variables (between a dependent variable and one or more independent variables).

Q: Define linear regression.

ONE-LINER QUESTIONS

Ans: Standard method for determining whether two variables are correlated or not.

Q: Define "coefficient of correlation".
Ans: This is indicative of the degree of correlation between the two variables, X and Y. The symbol denoting coefficient of correlation is r. Correlation coefficients vary between –1 and +1. A value of 1 is indicative of perfect correlation, whereas the value of 0 indicates no correlation at all.

Q: What is t-tests?
Ans: t-Tests is used for comparing the means of two groups from a single nominal variable, using means from an interval variable to see whether the groups are different groups or not.
For example, do patients with menorrhagia who are treated with tranexamic acid have a better quality of life in comparison to those who are not given this therapy?

Q: Define Chi-Square test.
Ans: 1. Used for evaluation of nominal data only
2. Any number of groups
3. Tests to see whether two nominal variables are independent or not. For example, testing the efficacy of a new drug by comparing the number of recovered patients given the drug with those who are not.

Q: What is a parametric test?
Ans: Parametric test is a statistical test that makes assumptions about the parameters (defining properties) of the population distribution(s) from which one's data are drawn.

Q: Give examples of parametric test.
Ans: Student's t-test and analysis of variance (ANOVA)

Q: What is a non-parametric test?
Ans: Non-parametric test is a statistical test that makes no such assumptions.

Q: Give an example of non-parametric test.

Ans: Mann-Whitney U-test and Wilcoxon signed rank test

Q: Which types of tests are preferred: parametric tests or non-parametric tests?
Ans: Parametric tests are preferred over the non-parametric tests because fewer observations are required to provide evidence in favour of the hypothesis if it is true.

Q: Which non-parametric test ranks the observations in the order of size and compares the proportions, which fall above and below the median value for each of the groups in question?
Ans: Mann-Whitney U test

Q: In which cases non-parametric tests and parametric tests employed?
Ans: *Non-parametric tests*: Employed in cases with sample size less than 15 observations, unlikely to have a normal distribution.
Parametric tests: In cases with more than 20 observations, with the data following a normal distribution.

Q: When does the odds ratio (OR) approximate the risk ratio (RR)?
Ans: When the disease being studied is rare.

Q: What is the correct formula to calculate the positive predictive value (if TP = true positive; FP = false positive; TN = true negative; FN = false negative)?
Ans: TP/(TP + FP)

Q: How to calculate standard error of the mean?
Ans: $SEM = SD/\sqrt{n}$

Q: What is the confidence interval of the range of one standard deviation (SD) above and one SD below the mean?
Ans: 68.2%

Q: What is prevalence?
Ans: The prevalence is the proportion of people in the entire population who are found to be with a disease at a certain point in time.

ONE-LINER QUESTIONS

Q: What are the features of prevalence rate of a disease?
Ans: 1. It can be used to determine the health needs of a community.
2. It can be estimated from a cross-sectional study.
3. It is dependent on the duration of illness and incidence of the disease.
4. It measures all the current cases in the community.

Q: What is incidence of the condition?
Ans: It is the number of newly diagnosed cases of the condition over a specific time period.

Q: What does incidence specify?
Ans: It tells how common a situation is.

Q: How many indices are employed for evaluating a clinical diagnostic test?
Ans: Four indices: sensitivity, specificity, positive predictive value, and the negative predictive value

Q: What is specificity of a test?
Ans: It is the probability of a negative test given the absence of the condition.

Q: How is disease specificity calculated?
Ans: Specificity is equal to true negatives/ (true negatives + false positives)

Q: What is sensitivity of a test?
Ans: It is the probability of the test being positive in somebody with the condition. It indicates the proportion of individuals with positive screening tests that actually have the disease.

Q: How is sensitivity calculated?
Ans: Sensitivity is equal to true positives/ (true positives + false negatives)

Q: What is positive predictive value?

Ans: It is the probability of having a condition if the test is positive. It is the probability of an event in the active group divided by the probability of the event in the control group.

Q: How is positive predictive value calculated?
Ans: It is calculated as follows: Positive predictive value = true positive/true positive + false positive

Q: Define negative predictive value.
Ans: It is defined as the proportion of individuals with negative tests that are free of the condition. It is the probability that the person who is test negative is actually a true negative.

Q: How is Negative predictive value calculated?
Ans: Negative predictive value = true negative/true negative + false negative

Q: Define variable.
Ans: It is defined as a value or a characteristic that can be changed.

Q: Which variable can take on only a certain number of values?
Ans: Discrete variable

Q: Which variables do not change with time and circumstance (e.g. gender and ethnicity)?
Ans: Discrete variable

Q: Define continuous variable.
Ans: These are variables, which can take up an infinite number of values. They change with time and circumstances.

Q: What type of variable is body mass index (BMI)?
Ans: Continuous

Q: What types of variables are blood pressure, height, weight and plasma concentrations
Ans: Continuous variable

Q: What is reliability of a test?

ONE-LINER QUESTIONS

Ans: It is the ability of a test to produce the same result when repeated under identical conditions.

Q: Define relative risk.
Ans: The ratio of the risk of disease in subjects with a given characteristic compared with those without that characteristic.

Q: What is confounding factor?
Ans: It is a factor, which is associated with both the exposure and the outcome under scrutiny.

Q: What is null hypothesis and alternative hypothesis?
Ans: Null hypothesis states that there is no difference between the two sets of data.
Alternative hypothesis states that there is a difference between the two groups.

Q: How is 95% CI calculated?
Ans: It is calculated as the mean± 1.96 times the standard error of the mean (SEM) for population greater than 30.

Q: What is the commonly used CI in the research studies and why?
Ans It is 95% CI because this corresponds to the P value of 0.05.

Q: Ninety-five percent CIs can be used for which type of data: distributional or distribution-free data?
Ans: Both distributional and distribution-free data

Q: What value of probability (P) is traditionally considered as the cut-off point for statistical significance?
Ans: P value of 0.05

Q: What P value is considered non-random or statistically significant?
Ans: P value of 0.05 or below

Q: What does P value of 0.01 implies?

Ans: It implies that the observation would be seen to occur by chance in 1 out of 100 occasions.

Q: Define statistical power of the study.
Ans: It is the ability of the study to detect a statistically significant difference between the two groups (i.e. if the difference really existed).

Q: How is power of a study related to sample size?
Ans: Power of a study increases with the increasing sample size.

Q: Which is the most commonly used type of distribution in medical statistics?
Ans: Normal or Gaussian distribution

Q: Which type of distribution forms the basis for the Student's t-test?
Ans: t distribution

Q: Which type of curve is generated if Gaussian distribution is plotted in terms of probability?
Ans: Bell-shaped curve

Q: Which test is the standard method for comparing distributions, e.g. between the observed and expected frequency of a given event?
Ans: Chi-squared test

Q: Which test is a standard test for comparing the difference between the two means?
Ans: Student's t-test

Q: Which test is the standard method for comparing the size of variance?
Ans: f-test

Q: Which parameters are most commonly used while summarising the skewed data and normally distributed data?
Ans: *When summarising skewed data*: the median and the interquartile range

ONE-LINER QUESTIONS

While summarising the normally distributed data: the mean and the standard deviation

Q: Which is the most appropriate measure in skewed data?
Ans: The geometric mean

Q: Which symbol denotes mean (the average of the data)?
Ans: The Greek letter mu, μ

Q: Which mean is preferred in normal statistics: arithmetic mean or geometric mean?
Ans: The arithmetic mean (as it generally represents the average)

Q: How is arithmetic mean calculated?
Ans: By using sum of the values [(a1+ ... +aN)/N]

Q: How is geometric mean calculated?
Ans: It is calculated as the nth root of the product of n numbers [n√(a1.a2.a3....aN)].

Q: Define median.
Ans: The median is the middle observation value. So, half the observations lie above this value and the other half lies below it.

Q: Define "mode".
Ans: Mode refers to the most frequently encountered value and in a normally distributed data coincides with the mean and median values.

Q: How is range calculated?
Ans: It is calculated by subtracting the lowest value from the highest value.

Q: What is an indication of variability of the observations?
Ans: Variance

Q: How is variance calculated?

Ans: To calculate the variance, each observation is subtracted from the mean, squared, added-up and divided by the number of observations minus one.

Q: Which is the standard method for determining whether two variables are correlated or not.
Ans: Linear regression

Q: What is the symbol denoting coefficient of correlation?
Ans: r

Q: Define standard error of mean.
Ans: It can be defined as the standard deviation of the sampling distribution of a statistical measurement, most commonly mean.

Q: How is standard deviation calculated?
Ans: This can be calculated as standard deviation divided by $\sqrt{n}$ or $\sqrt{n-1}$.

Q: What is odds ratio?
Ans: This can be defined as the ratio of the number of subjects classified in one category to the number of subjects classified in another category.

Q: What are the two most common types of bias encountered in the epidemiological studies?
Ans: The selection bias and the responder or the observer bias

Q: What is the best way for reducing the selection bias at the time of investigating the impact of treatment on the disease?
Ans: Using randomised controlled trials

Q: How does observer bias occurs?
Ans: It occurs when the investigator is aware of the disease status, treatment group, or outcome of the study.

Q: What are features of double blind study?
Ans: (1). Neither the study participants nor the person giving the treatment knows which treatment a particular subject is receiving.

ONE-LINER QUESTIONS

(2). Helps in alleviating potential bias through randomisation of patients to the drug or placebo without either the doctor or the patient knowing which agent is being used. (3). Both the researchers and the study participants are "blind" to which subject is receiving what type of treatment during the study. This method helps researchers get more accurate results from their research.

Q: What are features of placebo?
Ans: 1. Associated with placebo (psychological) effect
2. Should be identical in appearance to the drug being studied
3. Placebo studies are undertaken in patients with cancer.
4. Pharmacologically inert
5. Best administered by a person who is unaware of the drug's identity

Q: What are features of single blind study?
Ans: (1). Patient does not know which arm of therapy they are receiving. However, the investigator does have this information. (2). Patients are randomised by the investigators to receive either the drug or the placebo. (3). The patients are unaware regarding the kind of treatment they would receive.

Q: What are features of randomised controlled trials?
Ans: 1. Used for investigating the effects of therapies and interventions in the course of a particular treatment
2. Subjects with a particular condition who meet the inclusion criteria are included in study.
3. Subjects are randomly allocated to either receive treatment or some form of control (either no treatment or the current, "gold standard" treatment).
4. A computer program is used for randomising the data in different participating centres.
5. Various participating centres are linked with telephone services to request the randomisation procedure.

Q: What is the main advantage of the randomised control trial?
Ans: It is the concealment of the treatment allocation and thus minimisation of the selection bias and low chances of confounding.

Q: Define meta-analysis.
Ans: Meta-analysis is a common way of assessing the effect of treatment or the potential risks of treatment by reviewing and assessing all the data published in the medical literature to test the effectiveness of the results.

ONE-LINER QUESTIONS
CHAPTER 11
Pharmacology

Q: How is opioid toxicity monitored?
Ans: Respiratory rate

Q: What is the oestrogens sequence according to increasing efficacy?
Ans: Oestriol (E3)-Oestrone (E1)-Oestradiol (E2)

Q: Which drug for urinary tract infection is not safe in 3rd trimester?
Ans: Nitrofurantoin

Q: Which drug causes lactic acidosis?
Ans: Metformin

Q: Which antithyroid drug is used in pregnancy?
Ans: Propylthiouracil (PTU)

Q: Which drug is used for the treatment of benzodiazepines poisoning?
Ans: Flumazenil

Q: Which is the nephrotoxic antibiotic?
Ans: Aminoglycosides

Q: Which is the drug of choice for rheumatoid arthritis?
Ans: Azathioprine

Q: Which antimetabolite is the prodrug for 6-mercaptopurine?
Ans: Azathioprine

Q: What is the amphipathic criterion of a drug to cross placenta?
Ans: Lipid solublity

Q: What is the mode of action of vincristine?
Ans: Inhibits function of microtubules

Q: What is the drug of choice for the treatment of MRSA?
Ans: Vancomycin

Q: Which is the most common anomaly caused by warfarin?
Ans: Nasal hypoplasia

Q: Which cytokine II inhibits HPV replication?
Ans: Interferon

Q: What is the mechanism of action of hydralazine?
Ans: Direct acting smooth muscle relaxant (vasodilation)

Q: Which receptor is responsible for the action of midazolam, an effective anxiolytic drug?
Ans: GABA

Q: Mifepristone is a drug used in medical termination of pregnancy. What is the mode of action of mifepristone?
Ans: Progesterone antagonist

Q: Why is Suxamethonium not able to readily cross the placenta?
Ans: High degree of ionisation

Q: Nifedipine belongs to which class of drugs?
Ans: Calcium channel blockers

Q: Which cytokines are secreted by virally infected host cells and stimulates uninfected neighbouring cells to synthesize antiviral proteins?
Ans: Interferons alpha and beta (IFN α and IFN β)

Q: Lithium therapy during pregnancy increases the risk of congenital anomalies in which organ?
Ans: Heart

Q: What is the most common type of neoplasm occurring in the female genital tract of an 18-year-old girl whose mother was treated with diethylstilbestrol during pregnancy?

ONE-LINER QUESTIONS

Ans: Clear cell carcinoma of the vagina

Q: What is the mechanism of action of clomiphene citrate?
Ans: Selective oestrogen receptor modulator

Q: What is the mechanism of action of neostigmine?
Ans: Anticholinesterase

Q: In which cell organelle does phase I reactions occur?
Ans: Endoplasmic reticulum

Q: On which receptor does labetalol acts?
Ans: Alpha and beta adrenergic receptors

Q: What does warfarin acts against?
Ans: Prothrombin

Q: Oxytocin cannot be administrated by oral route due to which reason?
Ans: Oxytocin is destroyed by gastric juice.

Q: Which drugs is used to suppress lactation postpartum in mother who suffers from stillbirth?
Ans: Cabergoline

Q: What is the main action of COCPs?
Ans: Inhibit ovulation

Q: Where do phase II reactions occur?
Ans: Cytoplasm

Q: Which drugs may reduce the efficacy of the OCP?
Ans: Ampicillin, carbamazepine, rifampicin and phenytoin, tetracyclines, and metronidazole

Q: Which drug combinations must be avoided to prevent development of adverse reactions?

Ans: 1. Combination of sildenafil and isosorbide mononitrate (may cause a profound hypotension)
2. Combination of statin therapy and fibrates are sometimes used in cases of hyperlipidaemia (may cause myositis)
3. Metronidazole in combination with alcohol (produces an antabuse/disulfiram effect associated with nausea/vomiting and flushing)

Q: What effect beta-sympathomimetic drugs exert on mean blood pressure and why?
Ans: These drugs exert little or no effect on the mean blood pressure. It is because the increase in blood pressure resulting from increased heart rate and contractility is counteracted by the decrease in total peripheral resistance due to vasodilation in blood vessels perfusing skeletal muscle.

Q: To which class of drugs ephedrine, amphetamine, and isoprenaline belong?
Ans: Sympathomimetic amines

Q: What type of amine is Histamine ?
Ans: Vasoactive

Q: What are the adverse effects of beta sympathomimetic drugs?
Ans: Uterine relaxation, vasodilation, bronchial relaxation, intestinal and genitourinary wall relaxation, cardiac stimulation, glycogenolysis, renin release, gluconeogenesis, lipolysis, etc.

Q: Clonidine is an alpha adrenergic receptor ?
Ans: agonist

Q: Why should clonidine be withdrawn slowly?
Ans: Because sudden withdrawal can cause a severe hypertensive crisis.

Q: Why propranolol is effective in treatment of angina?
Ans: Through antagonism of the beta-1 receptors, propranolol has negative chronotropic effects on the heart causing reduced

myocardial oxygen consumption and so it is an effective treatment in angina.

Q: Which benzodiazepines are long-acting hypnotics?
Ans: Nitrazepam and flurazepam. Commonly used for early morning insomnia

Q: Which benzodiazepines are short-acting hypnotics?
Ans: Oxazepam, temazepam, and triazolam

Q: Which benzodiazepines are anxiolytics?
Ans: Diazepam, chlordiazepoxide, and lorazepam

Q: Are benzodiazepines prescribed during pregnancy?
Ans: They should be avoided in late pregnancy. Short acting benzodiazepines are preferable during pregnancy.

Q: What are the side-effects produced by antipsychotic drugs?
Ans: Hyperprolactinaemia and extrapyramidal side effects (e.g. malignant neuroleptic syndrome, tardive Parkinsonism, acute muscular dystonias, akathisia, dyskinesia, etc.).
Anticholinergic side effects: Dry mouth, blurring of vision, constipation, etc.

Q: By which mechanism monoamine oxidase inhibitors elevate the mood?
Ans: These drugs inhibit the enzyme MAO (monoamine oxidase) thus resulting in mood elevation. MAO is a mitochondrial enzyme involved in the oxidative deamination of biogenic amines.

Q: What is the impact of tricyclic antidepressants, if given in the third trimester?
Ans: Tricyclic antidepressants may cause tachycardia and irritability in the neonate especially if taken in the third trimester (especially imipramine).

Q: List the drugs included as selective serotonin reuptake inhibitors.

Ans: These include drugs like fluoxetine, citalopram, fluvoxamine, paroxetine, sertraline, escitalopram, and dapoxetine.

Q: Which SSRI is not recommended in children?
Ans: Use of fluoxetine

Q: Which SSRI is recommended for treatment of premature ejaculation?
Ans: Fluoxetine

Q: Which drugs are included in atypical antidepressants?
Ans: Trazodone, mianserin, tianeptine, mirtazapine, bupropion, and amineptine

Q: Which drugs are included in serotonin and noradrenaline reuptake inhibitors?
Ans: Venlafaxine and duloxetine

Q: Why NSAIDs are avoided during the third trimester?
Ans: Due to the theoretical risk of premature closure of ductus arteriosus and unproven concerns of teratogenicity

Q: Which analgesic is used in labour to block the sympathetic response to pain?
Ans: Pethidine

Q: Why methadone is not used during pregnancy?
Ans: Because it has a long elimination half-life of 23 hours in the foetus

Q: Which analgesic is extensively used analgesic drug during pregnancy and is safe during pregnancy and lactation?
Ans: Codeine

Q: What are features of infants of opiate-abusing mothers?
Ans: 1. Likely to be small for gestational age
2. Incidence of SIDS is significantly higher
3. Opiate withdrawal leads to an increased metabolic rate

ONE-LINER QUESTIONS

Q: Why nalorphine is not clinically useful?
Ans: Due to a high incidence of dysphoria

Q: Which biguanide (therapy) may help improve the rate of conception, oligomenorrhea, and hirsutism?
Ans: Metformin therapy

Q: Why metformin should be used with caution in patients with renal impairment?
Ans: It does not cause renal impairment. But should be used with caution because of risk of lactic acidosis. It should not be used in subjects whose creatinine clearance is above 130 mmol/l or heart failure.

Q: Which drug (belonging to the sulphonylurea class of hypoglycaemic drugs) is used for treating type 2 diabetes?
Ans: Chlorpropamide

Q: Which diuretics are known as high ceiling diuretics? Give examples.
Ans: Loop diuretics. They include bumetanide, furosemide, and torsemide.

Q: What is the primary site of action of thiazide diuretics?
Ans: Their primary site of action is the cortical diluting segment or the early distal tubule.

Q: What is the mechanism of action of thiazide diuretics?
Ans: They act by inhibiting the Na^+-Cl^- symport. It can cause hyperuricaemia, hypokalaemia, hypochloremic alkalosis, and hyperglycaemia.

Q: What is the primary site of action of potassium sparing diuretics?
Ans: These drugs act on the distal convoluted tubule.

Q: What is the mechanism of action of potassium sparing diuretics?

Ans: These drugs act on the DCT through various mechanisms, inhibiting the loss of potassium in exchange for sodium. These drugs can cause potassium retention and oestrogenic side effects.

Q: Why is metoclopramide particularly used before anaesthesia?
Ans: Metoclopramide has a central phenothiazine-like effect (sedative drug) with gastric emptying, so it is particularly used before anaesthesia.

Q: Which drug causes increased gastrointestinal motility, increases sphincter tone, and also has central antiemetic actions mediated through dopaminergic receptors?
Ans: Metoclopramide

Q: To which class of antiemetic agent does meclozine (meclizine) belong?
Ans: H1 antihistaminics

Q: Which antiemetic is used for the prevention of nausea and vomiting in Parkinson's patients treated with apomorphine?
Ans: Domperidone

Q: What are the contraindications of emetics?
Ans: Central nervous system (CNS) stimulant drug poisoning; corrosive (acid, alkali) poisoning; kerosene (petroleum) poisoning; unconscious patient; and morphine or phenothiazine poisoning

Q: What are tocolytic drugs?
Ans: Drugs which inhibit the uterine contractions

Q: Name the tocolytic drugs.
Ans: Glyceryl trinitrate (GTN); ritodrine; alcohol; nifedipine; magnesium sulphate; salbutamol; and non-steroidal anti-inflammatory drugs (NSAIDs)

Q: Where is oxytocin synthesized and stored?
Ans: It is synthesised within the nerve cell bodies in supraoptic and paraventricular nuclei of hypothalamus and stored in the posterior pituitary.

ONE-LINER QUESTIONS

Q: What is the action of oxytocin on uterus?
Ans: Oxytocin has uterotonic action. It helps in increasing the force and frequency of uterine contractions.

Q: What is the action of oxytocin on non-pregnant uterus, pregnant uterus, and puerperium?
Ans: Non-pregnant uterus and that during early pregnancy is rather resistant to oxytocin; sensitivity increases progressively in the third trimester, with a sharp increase occurring near term. The sensitivity quickly falls during the puerperium.

Q: What is the action of oxytocin on breast tissues?
Ans: In the breast tissues, oxytocin contracts the myoepithelial cells of mammary alveoli, thereby forcing the milk into the bigger milk sinusoids, resulting in the "milk ejection reflex" or the "let-down reflex".

Q: Which drug is recommended as the first-line drug in active management of third stage of labour? Why?
Ans: Oxytocin. Because of its short half-life and good intensity of action. Its action can be quickly terminated and it does not cause contraction of the lower segment.

Q: What dose of syntocinon is required to induce labour at term?
Ans: 0.5–15 mU/min

Q: What is the drug of choice for inducing and augmenting labour?
Ans: Oxytocin

Q: Why is oxytocin usually preferred over ergometrine/PGs for inducing and augmenting labour?
Ans: 1. Intensity of oxytocin action can be controlled and be quickly terminated.
2. When used in low concentrations, oxytocin allows normal relaxation in between uterine contractions. So the foetal oxygenation is not compromised.

3. The lower uterine segment is not contracted, so foetal descent is not affected.
4. Uterine contractions are consistently augmented.

Q: What are adverse effects of using oxytocin?
Ans: 1. Strong uterine contractions
2. Tachysystole/uterine hyperstimulation
3. Maternal cardiovascular side effects: increase in the heart rate, systemic venous return and cardiac output, cardiac arrhythmias, premature ventricular contractions, etc.
4. Water intoxication: It may manifest in the form of symptoms of hyponatraemia such as confusion, coma, convulsions, congestive cardiac failure, and death.
5. Hypotension
6. It can result in foetal side effects (bradycardia, neonatal jaundice, low APGAR score, etc.)

Q: What are relative contraindications of oxytocin?
Ans: Previous uterine scar; vertex not fixed in the pelvis; unfavourable cervix; breech presentation; hydramnios; and multiple pregnancy

Q: What are indications of using Methergine?
Ans: 1. Prophylaxis and treatment of severe atonic PPH
2. Active management of third stage of labour
3. Following LSCS/hysterectomy, to facilitate uterine contractions

Q: What is the dose of Methergine for controlling atonic PPH as well as following the delivery of anterior shoulder in cases of normal vaginal delivery (active management of third stage of labour)?
Ans: 0.2 mg intramuscularly or intravenously stat

Q: What is the composition of Syntometrine?
Ans: It is a combination of ergometrine maleate 500 micrograms plus syntocinon 5 units in 1 ml.

Q: What are contraindications of Ergometrine?
Ans: Severe pre-eclampsia; suspected multifoetal pregnancy; eclampsia; and Rh-negative mothers

ONE-LINER QUESTIONS

Q: Name some antiprotozoal agents.
Ans: Chloroquine, pyrimethamine, metronidazole, diloxanide, etc.

Q: Name some anthelmintic agents.
Ans: Mebendazole, pyrantel, niclosamide, diethylcarbamazine, etc.

Q: Define bacteriostatic antibiotic and bactericidal antibiotic.
Ans: Bacteriostatic antibiotic: Biological or chemical agent that stops bacteria from reproducing or inhibits their growth, while not necessarily killing them otherwise.
Bactericidal antibiotic: Biological or chemical agent which kills the bacteria.

Q: Define beta-lactam antibiotics. Name two major types of antibiotics belonging to this group.
Ans: This is a group of antibiotics having a beta-lactam ring. Two antibiotics are penicillins and cephalosporins.

Q: What leads to penicillin resistance?
Ans: Penicillin resistance is usually due to production of altered penicillin-binding proteins or beta-lactamases which break the beta lactam ring and inactivate the drug.

Q: Which is the most powerful penicillin and the drug of choice for sensitive organisms?
Ans: Penicillin-G (PnG)

Q: What is the composition of Co-amoxiclav?
Ans: Co-amoxiclav consists of amoxicillin and the beta-lactamase inhibitor clavulanic acid.

Q: From where are cephalosporins, a group of semisynthetic antibiotics derived ?
Ans: "Cephalosporin-C" obtained from a fungus *Cephalosporium*.

Q: What is the main adverse effect related with cephalosporins?
Ans: The risk of drug allergy

Q: What is the distinctive feature of the fourth generation cephalosporin compounds?
Ans: It is non-susceptibility of this group of drugs to inducible chromosomal beta-lactamases as well as high potency against Enterobacteriaceae and spectrum of activity resembling the third generation compounds.

Q: Sulphonamides are structural analogues of?
Ans: PABA (p-aminobenzoic acid)

Q: What is the side effect of sulphonamides in newborn?
Ans: Kernicterus may precipitate in the newborn, especially the premature ones (as blood-brain barrier is more permeable).

Q: What is the composition of cotrimoxazole?
Ans: The fixed dose combination of trimethoprim and sulphamethoxazole is called cotrimoxazole.

Q: How does cotrimoxazole acts?
Ans: It acts via inhibition of folic acid synthesis.

Q: Name the diseases for which tetracyclines are specifically indicated?
Ans: Brucellosis, chlamydial, and rickettsial infections

Q: What are side effects of tetracycline use?
Ans: 1. Damage to the developing bones and teeth
2. Doxycycline can result in photosensitivity
3. Fatty infiltration of liver and jaundice
4. Oxytetracyclines can precipitate acute hepatic necrosis.
5. If administered from midpregnancy to 5th month of extrauterine life, it can affect the deciduous teeth.
6. If administered between 3 months and 6 years of age, it can affect the crown of permanent anterior dentition.
7. If administered during late pregnancy or childhood, it can cause temporary suppression of the bone growth.

Q: What type of antibiotic is chloramphenicol ?

ONE-LINER QUESTIONS

Ans: Broad-spectrum

Q: Which is the most important cause of aplastic anaemia, agranulocytosis, thrombocytopenia, or pancytopenia?
Ans: Chloramphenicol

Q: What is the effect of administration of chloramphenicol on infants and foetuses?
Ans: It can cause "grey baby syndrome" when administered to the infants, but does not harm the foetuses.

Q: What is the drug of choice for pertussis prophylaxis?
Ans: Erythromycin

Q: What is the main side effect which can occur with nitrofurantoin?
Ans: Development of pulmonary infiltration

Q: Why lincosamides are used for the treatment of osteomyelitis?
Ans: Because lincosamides are particularly concentrated in bones, so they are used for treatment of osteomyelitis

Q: Name the first generation fluoroquinolones.
Ans: Norfloxacin, ciprofloxacin, ofloxacin, and pefloxacin

Q: Name the second generation fluoroquinolones.
Ans: The second generation fluoroquinolones include drugs like gemifloxacin, levofloxacin, moxifloxacin, lomefloxacin, etc.

Q: Streptomycin is mainly reserved for the treatment of which disease?
Ans: Tuberculosis

Q: What is mode of administration of aminoglycosides?
Ans: 1. They cannot be administered orally as they are not absorbed from the gut. They are administered through parenteral route (usually via intravenous route).
2. Tobramycin can be given by a nebuliser.
3. Neomycin ointment can be used for skin infection.

Q: Which drug can cause plasma concentration-dependent nerve deafness that may be permanent?
Ans: Vancomycin

Q: What is "Red man syndrome"?
Ans: Rapid IV injection of vancomycin causes a syndrome, known as the "Red man syndrome". This is associated with chills, fever, urticaria, and intense flushing.

Q: Name the diseases for which Metronidazole (flagyl) is the treatment of choice?
Ans: *Trichomonas* and bacterial vaginosis

Q: Which drug can cause a "disulfiram-like" reaction when taken with alcohol?
Ans: Metronidazole (flagyl)

Q: How are alpha-interferon, beta-interferon, and gamma-interferon produced?
Ans: *Alpha-interferon*: Produced by unstimulated T cells and monocytes
Beta-interferon: Produced by stimulated epithelial cells in infected organs and by fibroblasts in tissue culture
Gamma-interferon: Produced by sensitised T cells

Q: Which drug is used in the treatment of HIV?
Ans: Zidovudine. It does not eliminate the HIV virus. It only reduces the HIV-related mortality rate and the incidence and severity of opportunistic infections.

Q: Which enzyme metabolises acyclovir to acyclovir triphosphate?
Ans: Herpes simplex specified enzyme (thymidine kinase)

Q: Which antifungal agents are topically used for vaginal infections?
Ans: Polyenes and imidazoles

Q: Which is the first orally effective broad-spectrum antifungal drug, useful in both dermatophytosis and deep mycosis?

ONE-LINER QUESTIONS

Ans: Ketoconazole

Q: What are the adverse effects of ketoconazole?
Ans: It decreases androgen production from testes, and displaces testosterone from protein binding sites. Because of this, a reduction in androstenedione and testosterone levels and an increase in progesterone and 17-hydroxyprogesterone levels occurs.

Q: At which stage of cell cycle alkylating agents cause structural damage to chromosomes?
Ans: At the time of replication during interphase

Q: Name drugs which are platinum derivatives.
Ans: Cisplatin and carboplatin
Cisplatin: Metastatic testicular, ovarian carcinoma, malignancies of lung, bladder, oesophagus, stomach, liver, and head and neck
Carboplatin: Ovarian carcinoma of epithelial origin, squamous carcinoma of head and neck, small cell lung cancer, breast cancer, and seminoma

Q: Which drug is used for the treatment of Hodgkin and non-Hodgkin lymphomas? What is its route of administration?
Ans: Mustine (Nitrogen mustard). It can be given only by IV route because it is highly reactive and local vesicant; it is administered into the tubing of fast-running infusion.

Q: Which is the drug of choice for chronic myeloid leukaemia?
Ans: Busulphan

Q: Doxorubicin is used for treatment of which type of tumours?
Ans: Acute myeloid and lymphoblastic leukaemia as well as solid tumours, such as breast, thyroid, ovary, bladder and lung cancers, sarcomas, and neuroblastoma.

Q: Which drug is used as an adjuvant therapy of breast carcinoma, and treatment of gastroesophageal, pancreatic, hepatic and bladder carcinoma?
Ans: Epirubicin

Q: What is the mechanism of action of heparin?
Ans: It enhances antithrombin III activity, which in turn inhibits activated factors XII, XI, X, IX, and thrombin. It also activates lipoprotein lipase in plasma, lowering the plasma triglycerides and inhibiting platelet aggregation by fibrin.

Q: What are the side effects of heparin?
Ans: Haemorrhage, hypersensitivity reactions, and osteoporosis (after prolonged administration). In high dosage, it may have an antiplatelet effect.

Q: What is the use of 5-fluorouracil?
Ans: Its primary use is induction of remission in cases of acute myelogenous as well as lymphoblastic leukaemia in children and adults. It is also used for treatment of blast crisis in chronic myelogenous leukaemia and non-Hodgkin's lymphoma.

Q: What is route of administration of heparin and warfarin?
Ans: *Heparin*: Parenteral (IV, SC)
Warfarin: Oral

Q: How does warfarin and its congeners act as anticoagulants in vivo, not in vitro?
Ans: This is because they act indirectly by interfering with the synthesis of vitamin K dependent clotting factors in the liver.

Q: What is impact of exposure of warfarin in first, second, and third trimester?
Ans: *First trimester*: Embryopathy in 5–10% of pregnancies
Second and third trimester: Recurrent brain microhaemorrhages, resulting in optic atrophy, dorsal midline dysplasia, and mental retardation

Q: Why ACE inhibitors are not recommended in late pregnancy?
Ans: ACE inhibitors can cause intrauterine growth restriction (IUGR), oligohydramnios, and neonatal anuria. Renal failure and death may occur.

ONE-LINER QUESTIONS

Q: What is the primary site of action of alpha-methyldopa?
Ans: It is a central sympathomimetic agent, acting on the α-receptors in sympathetic nuclei within the medulla reducing sympathetic activity.

Q: Why alpha-methyldopa is contraindicated in puerperium?
Ans: It is contraindicated in the puerperium. Its adverse effects on the mother are somnolence or depression.

Q: Why Beta-adrenoceptor blocking drugs are contraindicated in pregnancy?
Ans: It causes intrauterine growth restriction when given from early pregnancy. This is mostly seen when treatment is started early in the second trimester. So, beta-blockers are best contraindicated during pregnancy, except for short-term treatment in the third trimester.

Q: Why labetalol is preferred antihypertensive drug in pregnancy?
Ans: Because of its alpha-blocking action, labetalol causes arteriolar vasodilatation and lowers peripheral resistance. It is used for treating severe hypertension and pre-eclampsia. It helps in lowering BP smoothly but rapidly, without causing tachycardia.

Q: What is the route of administration of labetalol?
Ans: It can be administered via oral/intravenous route.

Q: In which conditions labetalol is contraindicated?
Ans: Congestive heart failure; asthma, airway obstructive disease; third-degree, second-degree heart block, or moderate-to-severe-first-degree heart block; bradycardia; hypotension; and cardiogenic shock

Q: Why monitoring of antiepileptic drugs is required during pregnancy?
Ans: 1. These drugs are capable of crossing placenta.
2. They can cause major abnormalities such as orofacial and congenital heart defects, neural tube defects, foetal hydantoin syndrome, etc.

Q: Which antiepileptic drugs are safe during pregnancy?
Ans: Carbamazepine, phenytoin, and valproic acid

Q: What are contraindications of sodium valproate?
Ans: Active liver disease; family history of severe hepatic dysfunction; and porphyria

Q: What is the dose of bromocriptine?
Ans: It is administered orally. Dose should always be started at a low dose: 1.25 mg BD and then gradually increased till response occurs or until the side effects become limiting. Bromocriptine in the dosage of 2.5–10 mg/day is useful in most cases.

Q: From which compound is Bromocriptine derived?
Ans: 2-bromo-aergocryptine

Q: What are the uses of lidocaine?
Ans: It is used for nerve block, surface application, infiltration, epidural, spinal, and intravenous regional block anaesthesia.

Q: What are side effects of lidocaine?
Ans: Overdose of this drug causes cardiac arrhythmias, fall in BP, muscle twitching, convulsions, coma, and respiratory arrest.

Q: Which is the most commonly used induction agent?
Ans: Thiopentone

Q: What is the concentration of NO commonly used for providing analgesia in labour?
Ans: 50% concentration of NO

Q: Name the fast acting general anesthetic drugs.
Ans: Propofol; thiopentone sodium; methohexitone sodium; and etomidate

Q: Which is the most widely used volatile anaesthetic drug?
Ans: Isoflurane

ONE-LINER QUESTIONS

Q: Why epidural block is contraindicated in antepartum haemorrhage?
Ans: Due to the dual risk of hypotension

Q: What are skeletal muscle relaxants?
Ans: Drugs acting peripherally at neuromuscular junction/muscle fibre itself or centrally in the cerebrospinal axis to reduce muscle tone and/or cause paralysis.

Q: What is the order of paralysis in case of competitive (non-depolarising block)?
Ans: Fingers, eyes → limbs → neck, face → trunk →respiratory

Q: Give examples of depolarising blockers.
Ans: Succinylcholine (SCh, Suxamethonium), decamethonium

Q: Mention the clinical conditions which are known for prolonging or potentiating the non-depolarising neuromuscular blockade.
Ans: Hypermagnesaemia; hypokalaemia; hypocalcaemia; metabolic alkalosis; respiratory acidosis; and hypothermia

Q: Which is the most commonly used muscle relaxant for passing tracheal tube?
Ans: Succinylcholine

Q: Name the drugs causing hypothyroidism.
Ans: Butazolidin; sulphonylureas; amiodarone; lithium; cobalt; iodides; and antithyroid drugs

Q: What is mechanism of action of antithyroid drugs?
Ans: These drugs inhibit the synthesis of thyroid hormones (T4) by preventing iodination of tyrosine residues.

Q: Which drug is used in the treatment of thyrotoxicosis in pregnancy?
Ans: Carbimazole

Q: In which period of foetal development teratogenic influence is likely to be strongest?
Ans: In the period of early organogenesis

Q: Which drug is teratogenic in the first trimester? What abnormalities are caused by this drug?
Ans: Warfarin. It can cause abnormalities such as stippling of the epiphyses, chondrodysplasia punctate, intracerebral haemorrhage, nasal hypoplasia, and CNS abnormalities.

Q: Which disease is caused by maternal use of phenytoin during pregnancy? Define it.
Ans: Phenytoin can cause foetal hydantoin syndrome. Foetal hydantoin syndrome is a syndrome comprising of characteristic pattern of mental and physical birth defects.

Q: Which disease is caused by maternal use of quinine during pregnancy?
Ans: It causes blindness and deafness by causing hypoplasia of optic nerve.

Q: Treatment with which medicine is a recognized indication for termination of the pregnancy?
Ans: Isotretinoin

Q: List antibiotics which must be avoided during pregnancy.
Ans: Tetracycline, chloramphenicol, ciprofloxacin, aminoglycosides, cotrimoxazole, nitrofurantoin, trimethoprim, and metronidazole

Q: Which is the only hypotensive that is safe in all stages of pregnancy?
Ans: Methyldopa

Q: What are the maternal and foetal complications of alcohol consumption during pregnancy?
Ans: *Maternal complications*: Preterm labour, miscarriage, etc.
Foetal complications: Foetal alcohol syndrome; growth restriction; foetal alcohol spectrum disorders; and neurodevelopmental anomalies

ONE-LINER QUESTIONS

Q: Which is the most commonly used screening tool for detecting alcohol abuse in antenatal clinics?
Ans: T-ACE questionnaire (at some places CAGE questionnaire is also used)

Q: Name the blood tests which could be used to screen for alcohol abuse.
Ans: Gamma glutamyl transpeptidase (GGT) and carbohydrate-deficient-transferrin (CDT)

Q: What are the three characteristic facial dysmorphic features the individual to be diagnosed with FAS must exhibit?
Ans: (1) Smooth philtrum, (2) thin vermillion upper lip border, and (3) small palpebral fissures

Q: Name the drugs which are secreted into the breast milk but are undetectable in the baby.
Ans: Drugs which are bound to maternal proteins (e.g. warfarin) or those which are not absorbed from the baby's gut (e.g. aminoglycosides)

Q: Name the drugs which are secreted into the breast milk and reach the baby in sufficient amounts so as to cause harm.
Ans: Lithium, cytotoxics, laxatives, barbiturates, immunosuppressive drugs, etc.

Q: List the drugs which can be used during breastfeeding.
Ans: Propranolol, warfarin, ranitidine, angiotensin-converting enzyme (ACE) inhibitors, beta-blockers, methyldopa, nifedipine or labetalol

Q: What are the indications for use of clomiphene citrate?
Ans: 1. Women with unexplained fertility problems
2. Women in whom the cause of infertility is anovulation or anovulatory disturbances
3. Polycystic ovarian disease
4. Anovulatory dysfunctional uterine bleeding

5. Harvesting oocytes before an IVF cycle
6. Oligospermia (in males)

Q: What is dose of leuprolide?
Ans: Leuprolide is used in the dosage of a single monthly 3.75 mg depot injection given intramuscularly.

Q: Danazol is the derivative of which compound?
Ans: Ethinyl testosterone

Q: Which is a highly effective drug for treatment of endometriosis?
Ans: Danazol

Q: What are the contraindications for the use of danazol?
Ans: Epileptic seizures; breast cancer; pregnant and lactating women; porphyrias; impaired renal/hepatic/cardiac function; and undiagnosed abnormal uterine bleeding

Q: What is the dose of mifepristone for termination of pregnancy up to 7 weeks of gestation?
Ans: For termination of pregnancy up to 7 weeks of gestation, 600 mg of mifepristone can be administered in the form of a single oral dose.

Q: What type of compound is Clomiphene citrate?
Ans: Both oestrogen antagonist and agonist

Q: In standard protocol, what is the standard dose of CC?
Ans: It is 50 mg PO once a day for 5 days, starting on the days 3–5 of the natural spontaneous menstrual cycle (follicular phase) or after progestin-induced bleeding.

Q: What is recommendation of UK Committee on the safety of medicines (CSM) regarding usage of clomiphene?
Ans: The UK Committee on the safety of medicines (CSM) has recommended that clomiphene should not normally be used for longer than six cycles.

ONE-LINER QUESTIONS

Q: What is the difference between the menopause like state produced by use of LHRH analogues and the real menopause?
Ans: The real menopause is associated with high levels of FSH and LH. The difference between the menopause like state produced by use of these drugs and the real menopause is that analogues produce their effect by inducing very low levels of FSH and LH.

Q: What are the adverse effects caused by danazol?
Ans: The adverse effects caused by this drug are related to oestrogen deficiency and the androgenic effects.
Oestrogen deficiency: Headache, flushing, sweating, atrophic vaginitis, and breast atrophy
Androgenic effects: Acne, oedema, hirsutism, deepening of the voice, and weight gain

Q: What is the dose of mifepristone used for cervical ripening before attempting surgical abortion or induction of labour?
Ans:: Mifepristone is given in the dosage of 600 mg, 24–30 hours before attempting surgical abortion or induction of labour. It helps in cervical softening and the facilitation of the procedure of surgical abortion.

Q: What dose of mifepristone is used for postcoital/emergency contraception?
Ans:: Mifepristone in the dosage of 600 mg administered within 72 hours of intercourse

Q: What are the contraindications for use of mifepristone?
Ans: Adrenal failure; haemorrhagic disorders; presence of IUCD; ectopic pregnancy; inherited porphyrias; intake of anticoagulants; and long-term corticosteroid therapy

Q: Which drug is used in the treatment of acne and hirsutism in form of the OCP?
Ans: Cyproterone acetate (in form of dianette)

Q: Which drug is used in the treatment of incontinence?
Ans: Duloxetine

ONE-LINER QUESTIONS
CHAPTER 12
Obstetrics

Q: What does the quadruple test positive means?
Ans: Decreased alpha-foetoprotein (AFP), increased β-hCG, and decreased unconjugated E3 levels

Q: Which causes premature closure of ductus arteriosus?
Ans: Indomethacin

Q: What is the most common clinical presentation case of obstetric cholestasis?
Ans: Generalized pruritus with normal liver enzymes

Q: Which is the anticoagulant drug of choice during pregnancy?
Ans: Heparin

Q: Which is the antidiabetic drug of choice during pregnancy?
Ans: Insulin

Q: What is the most common cause for anaemia during pregnancy?
Ans: Iron deficiency anaemia

Q: Which vitamin deficiency is associated with megaloblastic anaemia?
Ans: Folic acid

Q: What is the commonest mechanism for spread of choriocarcinoma?
Ans: Hematogenous

Q: What is the best screening method for haemolytic anaemia?
Ans: Haemoglobin

Q: What is the period of gestation if CRL = 10 mm?
Ans: 7 weeks

Q: Which vitamin converts ferric into ferrous to aid iron absorption?
Ans: Vitamin C

Q: Which clinical parameter must be monitored when there is overdose of pethidine?
Ans: Respiratory rate

Q: What is the medical treatment of choice in cases of ectopic pregnancy?
Ans: Methotrexate

Q: Misoprostol is a commonly used drug in the medical treatment of miscarriage. What type of drug is misoprostol?
Ans: Prostaglandin E1

Q: Whenever the intestinal midgut loop fails to return from the umbilical cord into the abdominal cavity, the defect is known as which of the following?
Ans: Exompholos

Q: What is the most common congenital solid tumour of the newborn?
Ans: Sacrococcygeal teratoma

Q: Which ovarian tumour is associated with Meigs syndrome?
Ans: Fibroma

Q: What is the most abundant carbohydrate in the breast milk?
Ans: Lactose

Q: At what stage does the combined oral contraceptive pills are safe to use following evacuation of a complete hydatidiform mole?
Ans: Return of βhCG titre to normal

Q: What kind of delivery can be opted for, if CTG baseline <100, variability <5, no acceleration, and late deceleration for 20 min?
Ans: C-section

ONE-LINER QUESTIONS

Q: What is the location of epidural space?
Ans: Between the wall of vertebral cavity and dura mater

Q: Which hernia will be the result of small defect in lateral umbilical region due to regression of umbilical vein?
Ans: Gastroschisis

Q: What is the average duration of human pregnancy?
Ans: It is 280 days from the first day of the last menstrual period (LMP).

Q: What is Naegele's rule?
Ans: The expected date of delivery (EDD) is calculated using Naegele's rule. This rule states that the EDD is calculated by adding 9 calendar months and 7 days to the first day of the LMP (28-day cycle).

Q: What is a good indicator of the gestational age on ultrasound measurement?
Ans: Measurement of the sac size between 6 weeks and 8 weeks is a good indicator of the gestational age.

Q: Define stillbirth.
Ans: It can be defined as foetal death after 24 completed weeks of pregnancy.

Q: Define miscarriage.
Ans: It is the loss of the products of conception before the foetus attains viability (before 24 completed weeks of gestation).

Q: Define abortion.
Ans: It is the premature expulsion of the products of conception, either embryo or non-viable foetus from the uterus.

Q: What are the β-hCG levels for intrauterine pregnancies to be visible on transvaginal scan (TVS)?
Ans: β-hCG levels are greater than 1,000 IU/L.

Q: Define threatened abortion.
Ans: Type of abortion where the process of abortion has begun but has yet not progressed to a stage from where the recovery would be impossible.

Q: What are the features of threatened abortion?
Ans: 1. Bleeding before 20 weeks of gestation. It may be with or without pain.
2. Cervical os is closed.

Q: Which maternal investigations are required for the detection of diabetes mellitus (DM) following a term stillbirth?
Ans: Maternal glycosylated haemoglobin levels

Q: Which test helps in establishing the presence of foetal red blood cells and in quantitating the volume of foetomaternal transfusion?
Ans: Kleihauer blood test

Q: Which maternal investigations are done following a term stillbirth?
Ans: Kleihauer blood test; glycosylated haemoglobin; platelet count; blood pressure measurement; and antinuclear antibody estimation

Q: According to Abortion Act (1967) in the UK, what is the upper gestational age limit for medical termination of pregnancy?
Ans: Upper gestational age limit of 24 weeks. In case of foetal abnormality, no upper limit exists.

Q: What results in development of Hydatidiform mole?
Ans: It results from overproduction of the chorionic tissue, which is normally supposed to develop into the placenta.

Q: What is the appearance of uterus in case of Hydatidiform mole?
Ans: It may appear doughy in consistency due to lack of foetal parts and amniotic fluid.

Q: What is clinical presentation of Hydatidiform mole?
Ans: Passage of vesicles, hyperemesis, uterus large for dates, ovarian cysts, hyperthyroidism, early-onset pre-eclampsia, etc.

ONE-LINER QUESTIONS

Q: What is the ratio of a partial: complete mole?
Ans: It is less than 3:1.

Q: What are the findings on vaginal examination in case of Hydatidiform mole?
Ans: 1. Vaginal bleeding or passage of grapelike vesicles
2. Internal ballottement cannot be elicited due to lack of foetus
3. Unilateral or bilateral enlargement of the ovaries in the form of theca lutein cysts may be palpable.

Q: What is the genetic composition of complete mole?
Ans: Karyotype 46XX

Q: What is the genetic composition of partial mole?
Ans: Triploid karyotype 69XXY

Q: What is the aetiology of complete mole?
Ans: Duplication of the haploid sperm following fertilization of an "empty" ovum or dispermic fertilization of an "empty" ovum

Q: Name the causes where uterine size is larger than the dates.
Ans: Uterine fibroids/leiomyomas; polyhydramnios; foetal macrosomia; multiple births; and diabetes

Q: Which investigation is fundamental for the follow-up in case of Hydatidiform mole?
Ans: β-hCG assay. Because the level correlates well with the amount of residual tumour.

Q: What are the findings on Ultrasound of the pelvis in case of Hydatidiform mole?
Ans: 1. Blighted ovum may be observed.
2. Characteristic vesicular pattern, also known as "snowstorm appearance"
3. An enlarged uterine endometrial cavity containing homogeneously hyperechoic endometrial mass with innumerable anechoic cysts.

4. Presence of theca lutein cysts in the ovaries

Q: What are the two main treatment options in case of H. mole?
Ans: Suction evacuation and hysterectomy

Q: What is the recommendation of RCOG on suction evacuation of H. mole?
Ans: The RCOG advises that:
1. Syntocinon infusions should not be used until the uterus has been evacuated.
2. Prostaglandins should only be used, if syntocinon has failed.
3. Avoid mifepristone as it increases the sensitivity of the uterus to prostaglandins.

Q: What is the main complication associated with H. mole?
Ans: The main complication associated with H. mole is the risk of development of persistent gestational trophoblastic neoplasia (GTN).

Q: What is the ratio of transverse to anterior-posterior dimension of the gestational sac in case of partial mole?
Ans: There is an increase in the ratio of transverse to anterior-posterior dimension of the gestational sac to a value greater than 1.5.

Q: What are the diseases associated with the spectrum of gestational trophoblastic neoplasia or the persistent disease?
Ans: Placental site trophoblastic tumour (PSTT); invasive mole; choriocarcinoma; and epithelioid trophoblastic tumour

Q: Which is the most common site for metastasis in case of malignant GTD?
Ans: The lungs

Q: What are the findings on chest X-ray in case of metastatic disease?
Ans: On chest X-ray, the lungs may show presence of distinct nodules or cannon ball appearance.

ONE-LINER QUESTIONS

Q: Define the scoring system adopted by the WHO and FIGO for classification of gestational trophoblastic tumours.
Ans: According to the system adopted by the WHO and FIGO scoring system:
1. Low-risk group has a score of 0–6
2. Moderate-risk group has a score between 5 and 7
3. High-risk group will have a score of 7 or higher.

Q: What is the standard multi-agent chemotherapy regimen in high-risk group gestational trophoblastic tumours?
Ans: The standard multi-agent chemotherapy regimen in high-risk group is EMA/CO. In this regimen, the drugs (like etoposide, dactinomycin, and methotrexate) are alternated at weekly intervals with vincristine and cyclophosphamide.

Q: How does an invasive mole develops?
Ans: It is a histologically benign condition. It results because of the invasion of abnormal trophoblasts into the myometrium. It can also develop due to embolisation of molar tissue through pelvic venous plexus.

Q: Where is the site of development of placental site trophoblastic tumour (PSTT)?
Ans: Develops at placental implantation site

Q: What is the origin of placental site trophoblastic tumour?
Ans: These tumours usually originate from the intermediate trophoblastic cells.

Q: What is the most common site of implantation in ectopic pregnancy?
Ans: Most commonly (in about 95% of cases), the fertilised ovum gets implanted inside the fallopian tube.

Q: What are the other extrauterine locations where an ectopic pregnancy can get implanted?
Ans: Fallopian tube, ovary, abdomen, or the cervix

Q: What is the major cause of ectopic pregnancy?
Ans: Acute salpingitis

Q: What is the typical triad on history for ectopic pregnancy?
Ans: Bleeding, abdominal pain, and a positive urine pregnancy test

Q: What are the findings on vaginal examination in case of ectopic pregnancy?
Ans: 1. Vaginal bleeding
2. Uterine or cervical motion tenderness
3. The uterus may be slightly enlarged and soft.
4. An adnexal mass may be palpated.

Q: What is the treatment given to Rh-negative patients to prevent the occurrence of haemolytic disease of the newborn?
Ans: Rh-negative patients must be injected with 50 μg of anti-D immune globulins.

Q: What is Doughnut or Bagel sign?
Ans: In case of an ectopic pregnancy, on ultrasound examination, a thick, bright echogenic, ring-like structure is shown, which is located outside the uterus, having a gestational sac containing an obvious foetal pole, yolk sac, or both. This usually appears as an intact, well-defined tubal ring (Doughnut or Bagel sign).

Q: What are the ultrasonographic findings in case of a ruptured ectopic pregnancy?
Ans: Presence of free fluid or clotted blood in the cul-de-sac or in the intraperitoneal gutters

Q: What is pregnancy of unknown location?
Ans: In this condition, the pregnancy test is positive, but there are no signs of intrauterine or extrauterine pregnancy on the TVS.

Q: What is the protocol for the management of pregnancy of unknown location?
Ans: It usually comprises of β-hCG assays, serial scans, and measurements of progesterone levels.

ONE-LINER QUESTIONS

Q: What level of progesterone indicates failed pregnancy, miscarriage, or ectopic pregnancy?
Ans: Progesterone levels less than 20 nmol/L

Q: Define heterotopic pregnancy.
Ans: A rare complication of pregnancy where both intrauterine and extrauterine pregnancies (ectopic pregnancy) co-exist simultaneously.

Q: What are the ultrasound findings and levels of β-hCG in heterotopic pregnancy?
Ans: *β-hCG levels*: Normal
Ultrasound scan: Shows an intrauterine sac and eventually a viable intrauterine pregnancy.
Coexisting ectopic pregnancy may produce an adnexal mass and free fluid in the pouch of Douglas.

Q: What are the ultrasound findings and levels of β-hCG in "Pregnancy of unknown location"?
Ans: β-hCG levels greater than 1,500 IU/L, with no evidence of an intrauterine pregnancy on a transvaginal ultrasound scan.

Q: Define anaemia according to WHO and CDC.
Ans: *WHO*: Defines anaemia as presence of haemoglobin of less than 11 g/dL and haematocrit of less than 0.33 g/dL.
CDC, 1990: Defines anaemia as haemoglobin levels below 11 g/dL in the pregnant woman in first and third trimester and less than 10.5 g/dL in second trimester.

Q: What are the two most sensitive indices of iron deficiency?
Ans: Mean corpuscular volume and mean corpuscular haemoglobin concentration

Q: What is the WHO recommendation regarding iron supplementation?
Ans: The WHO recommendation: in countries with prevalence of anaemia less than 40%, universal iron supplementation comprising of 60 mg elemental iron and 400 µg of folic acid is recommended

once or twice daily for 6 months in pregnancy. This supplementation is continued for an additional 3 months post-partum in countries where prevalence is greater than 40%.

Q: By what amount requirement of iron is increased in pregnancy?
Ans: Increased iron requirement during pregnancy: 1,000 mg. Iron requirements in singleton pregnancy increase from about 2.5 mg per day in the first trimester to about 6.5 mg per day in the third trimester.

Q: What is the average daily requirement of iron in pregnant woman?
Ans: Approximately 4 mg on an average

Q: What are the findings on peripheral smear in iron deficiency anaemia?
Ans: 1. Microcytic and hypochromic cells
2. Anisocytosis (abnormal size of cells) in the form of microcytosis and/or poikilocytosis (abnormal shape of cells) in the form of pencil cells and target cells.
3. Presence of ring or pessary cells with central hypochromia

Q: What level of ferritin is diagnostic of iron deficiency?
Ans: A ferritin level less than 12 µg/L

Q: What are the main problems associated with the use of oral iron supplements?
Ans: Epigastric discomfort, anorexia, diarrhoea, nausea, etc.

Q: What haemoglobin level is considered as an indication for iron therapy in UK?
Ans: In the UK, haemoglobin level considered to be abnormal is less than 10.5 g/dL and can be considered as an indication for therapy.

Q: Why ferrous salts are more commonly used in iron therapy in pregnant woman?
Ans: Since ferrous salts are better absorbed than ferric, they are more commonly used.

ONE-LINER QUESTIONS

Q: What are the two most commonly used parenteral iron preparations?
Ans: Iron sorbitol citric acid complex (Jectofer) and iron dextran (Imferon)

Q: What are the complications due to anaemia in mother during antenatal period?
Ans: Placenta praevia, accidental haemorrhage, poor weight gain, preterm labour, PIH, eclampsia, premature rupture of membranes (PROM), etc.

Q: What are the risk factors for the development of megaloblastic anaemia?
Ans: Multiple pregnancies; epilepsy; high parity; low income; and patients with malabsorption

Q: What therapy helps in the prevention of neural tube defects during pregnancy?
Ans: Folate supplementation, 1 month before conception and then throughout the first trimester

Q: What results in sickle cell disease in pregnancy?
Ans: It results from an amino acid substitution of glutamine for valine on the beta globin chain of the haemoglobin molecule.

Q: Why is pre-pregnancy or first trimester screening recommended in cases of sickle cell disease?
Ans: By pre-pregnancy or first trimester screening, the couple can be advised on the possible risk of a serious haemoglobin defect in their offspring and subsequently counselled about prenatal diagnostic options.

Q: What is the birth weight of infants in case of intrauterine growth restriction?
Ans: Birth weight is below the 10th percentile of the average for the particular gestational age

Q: What are small for gestational age infants?

Ans: The infants who have failed to achieve a specific weight or biometric size in accordance with the gestational age. He/she may not be pathologically growth restricted.

Q: Is there any pathological process involved in IUGR?
Ans: The growth restriction is due to some pathological process (either intrinsic or extrinsic).

Q: Which are the foetal causes which results in IUGR?
Ans: Chromosomal abnormalities (trisomy 13, 16, 18, 21, etc.); multiple pregnancy; congenital malformations (e.g. congenital heart disease, renal agenesis, etc.); and chronic intrauterine infection (e.g. TORCH, congenital syphilis, viral, bacterial, protozoal, and spirochetal infections).

Q: Which are the placental causes which results in IUGR?
Ans: Marginal or velamentous cord insertion, chorioangioma, circumvallate placenta, placenta praevia, placental abruption, etc.

Q: What are the main risks associated with anti-epilepsy drugs?
Ans: Neural tube defects, facial clefts, and cardiac abnormalities

Q: In case of mother suffering from epilepsy, why mother is given vitamin K (10 mg daily) in the last month of pregnancy?
Ans: Most of the anti-epileptic drugs induce cytochrome P450 enzymes, which reduce vitamin K levels in mother and baby. A small risk of neonatal bleeding is also there.

Q: What is frequent complication (90%) of rheumatic valvular heart disorder during pregnancy?
Ans: Mitral stenosis

Q: Define gestational diabetes as per WHO.
Ans: Carbohydrate intolerance resulting in hyperglycaemia of variable severity with the onset or first recognition during pregnancy.

ONE-LINER QUESTIONS

Q: What is the difference in levels of maternal α-feto-protein and unconjugated oestriol in women with insulin-dependent DM and those without diabetes?
Ans: Women with insulin-dependent DM have significantly lower levels of maternal α-feto-protein and unconjugated oestriol in comparison to the women without diabetes.

Q: As per the National Institute for Health and Care Excellence (NICE) guidelines (2015), what should be HbA1c levels during pregnancy?
Ans: HbA1c levels should be below 6.5%. Women should be advised to avoid pregnancy if the HbA1c is greater than 10%.

Q: What is glucose challenge test?
Ans: It is a screening test for gestational diabetes. In this test, plasma blood glucose levels are measured 1 hour after giving 50 g glucose load to the woman (irrespective of the time of the day or last meal).

Q: In GCT, what value indicates high risk for development of gestational diabetes?
Ans: A value of 140 mg/dL or higher

Q: Mention high-risk cases in which the glucose testing must be performed.
Ans: 1. Body mass index (BMI) >30 kg/m^2
2. History of delivery of previous baby having a weight greater than 4.5 kg
3. History of gestational diabetes
4. First-degree relative with diabetes
5. Strong family history of type II DM
6. Ethnicity (origin in India, Pakistan, Bangladesh, Caribbean and Middle East)

Q: What should be fasting blood sugar levels and 1-hour postprandial levels during pregnancy?
Ans: Fasting blood sugar levels: Between 3.5 mmol/litre and 5.9 mmol/litre
One-hour postprandial levels: Less than 7.8 mmol/litre

Q: When should a pregnant woman with diabetic nephropathy be referred to a nephrologist?
Ans: If serum creatinine is abnormal (≥120 mmol/litre) or if total protein excretion exceeds 2 g/day

Q: What should be calories intake in case of gestational diabetes?
Ans: BMI 25.9–29.9 kg/m²: 25 kcal/kg/day or less
BMI 18.5–24.9 kg/m²: Approximately 30 Kcal/kg/day
BMI <18.5: 35–40 Kcal/kg/day
BMI 30.0–49.9: 20 Kcal/kg/day
BMI ≥50: 12 Kcal/kg/day

Q: What is alternative for women who are either unable to take insulin or are non-responsive to it?
Ans: Treatment with glyburide. Metformin, a biguanide compound (glucophage) may be considered as another option.

Q: Which insulin is used during pregnancy?
Ans: Isophane insulin (intermediate-acting insulin)

Q: What are the major changes related in thyroid function during normal pregnancy?
Ans: Increase in serum thyroxine-binding globulin (TBG) concentrations; stimulation of the thyrotropin receptor by chorionic gonadotropin; and TBG excess resulting in an increase in the concentration of both serum total thyroxine (T4) and triiodothyronine (T3) (whereas free serum T4 and T3 concentrations remain within normal range).

Q: Which is the commonest cause of thyrotoxicosis in pregnancy?
Ans: Grave's disease, which accounts for about 95% cases

Q: Which is the commonest cause of hypothyroidism in pregnancy?
Ans: Hashimoto's disease

Q: Define De Quervain's thyroiditis.

ONE-LINER QUESTIONS

Ans: It is an inflammatory thyroiditis, which can result in hypothyroidism. It is thought to be of viral origin and is the commonest cause of a painful thyroid.

Q: Which is the biggest problem related to hypothyroidism in pregnancy?
Ans: Congenital cretinism due to iodine deficiency

Q: In UK, which investigation is done for screening of hypothyroidism in all newborn babies?
Ans: Guthrie test. This is a heel prick bloodspot test.

Q: What is the value of TSH for the diagnosis of hyperthyroidism in pregnant women?
Ans: Serum TSH value less than 0.01 mU/litre and a high serum free T4 value

Q: What drugs are recommended for treatment of moderate to severe hyperthyroidism complicating pregnancy?
Ans: Thioamides [propylthiouracil (PTU), methimazole, and carbimazole] are recommended.

Q: What drugs are recommended for treatment of hypothyroidism complicating pregnancy?
Ans: Levothyroxine in the dosage of 1–2 µg/kg/day (approximately 100 µg/day)

Q: What is the biggest risk to the mother in case of hyperthyroidism during pregnancy?
Ans: Thyroid storm. This is rare condition. This can cause heart failure and death in up to 30% cases.

Q: What are characteristics of obstetric cholestasis?
Ans: 1. Presence of pruritus and abnormal liver function tests (LFT) that resolve during the puerperium
2. Intense pruritus often occurs on the palms and soles
3. Usually, there is no rash, unless one inflicted by scratching. If there is a rash, a dermatological opinion must be taken.

Q: Which parameter is widely used for the diagnosis of OC in the UK?
Ans: Elevated bile acids

Q: What are the complications during labour in case of multiple pregnancy?
Ans: Cord entanglement; foetal malpresentation; vasa praevia; cord prolapse; dysfunctional uterine contractions; premature separation of placenta, resulting in abruption placenta; post-partum haemorrhage; and increased operative interference

Q: What are the foetal complications specific to twin gestation?
Ans: Conjoined twins, discordant growth, twin-to-twin transfusion, acardiac twin or twin reversed arterial perfusion syndrome, etc.

Q: Which is the commonest type of hydramnios?
Ans: Mild to moderate severity

Q: Which parameter is the basis of ultrasound diagnosis of hydramnios?
Ans: The ultrasound diagnosis of hydramnios is based on the calculation of "amniotic fluid index" (AFI) or evaluation of the "deepest vertical pool" (DVP).

Q: Which investigation is accepted as the gold standard for diagnosis and monitoring of foetal anaemia?
Ans: Middle cerebral artery (MCA) velocimetry

Q: What are characteristics of pre-eclampsia?
Ans: High blood pressure (>140/90 mmHg) and proteinuria (>300 mg/dL or >1+ on the dipstick)

Q: during what period of gestation does pre-eclampsia develop and regress?
Ans: *Develops*: After the 20th week of pregnancy
Regresses: After the delivery (usually within the 12th post-partum week)

Q: What is clinical presentation of pre-eclampsia?

ONE-LINER QUESTIONS

Ans: 1. Presence of increased BP (>140/90 mmHg) after 20 weeks of gestation
2. Excretion of proteins exceeds 300 mg per 24 hours or there is persistent presence of the protein (30 mg/dL or 1+ dipstick) in a random urine sample
3. Oedema of hands and face
4. Headache, visual problems, epigastric or right upper quadrant abdominal pain, oliguria (urine volume <500 mL/24 hours)
5. Shortness of breath or dyspnea
6. Reduced foetal movements
7. Weight gain of more than 2 pounds per week or 6 pounds in a month
8. Placental insufficiency
9. Placental abruption and associated bleeding

Q: What are the features of Grade 3 hypertensive retinopathy?
Ans: Haemorrhages and exudates

Q: What is treatment of pre-eclampsia?
Ans: The most commonly used first-line drugs include hydralazine (for severe hypertension), alpha-methyldopa, labetalol, and nifedipine.

Q: Which drug is used mostly as standard in management of eclampsia and severe pre-eclampsia?
Ans: In the UK, magnesium sulphate has become a standard protocol for management of eclampsia and severe pre-eclampsia. A total dose of 14 g is administered in form of loading (4 g IV) and maintenance dose (5 g in each buttock by deep IM injection).

Q: What is the mode of delivery in case of pre-eclampsia?
Ans: As such, severe pre-eclampsia is not an indication for caesarean section. The mode of delivery can be aas follows:
Cervix is ripe: Labour can be induced by using intravenous oxytocin and artificial rupture of membranes (ARM).
Unfavourable cervix or other complications (e.g. breech presentation, foetal distress, etc.): Caesarean section may be required.

Q: Define eclampsia.
Ans: Onset of tonic-clonic convulsions in a pregnant patient with pre-eclampsia, usually occurring in the third trimester of pregnancy, intra-partum period, or more than 48 hours post-partum.

Q: What are symptoms of eclampsia?
Ans: 1. *Premonitory stage*: There is unconsciousness; twitching of the muscles of face, tongue and limbs; and rolling and fixation of eyeballs. Twitching starts from the face onto the extremities and soon involves the whole body.
2. *Tonic stage*: There is tonic spasm of the body muscles.
3. *Clonic stage*: There is alternate contraction and relaxation of the skeletal muscles.
4. *Coma*: This may be present for a brief period or may persist for a longer time.

Q: What is treatment of choice for convulsions in case of eclampsia?
Ans: Administration of magnesium sulphate

Q: Define hyperemesis gravidarum.
Ans: HG is occurrence of severe vomiting causing loss of greater than 5% of body weight.

Q: What are the features associated with hyperemesis gravidarum?
Ans: 1. Persistent vomiting is present.
2. Loss of weight
3. Ketosis
4. Dehydration
5. Disturbed electrolytes (low potassium and sodium, raised liver transaminases, low blood urea level, etc.)

Q: When does onset of hyperemesis gravidarum occurs?
Ans: Onset is in the first trimester

Q: What are the complications of hyperemesis gravidarum?
Ans: Wernicke's encephalopathy due to thiamine (vitamin B1) deficiency, deep vein thrombosis, pulmonary embolism, IUGR, hypokalaemia, hyponatraemia, Mallory-Weiss oesophageal tears, Korsakoff's psychosis, stillbirth, etc.

ONE-LINER QUESTIONS

Q: What conditions are screened in pre-implantation genetic screening?
Ans:
1. Used in women above 35 years of age, when semen has been obtained using intracytoplasmic sperm injection (ICSI) and when there are particular genetic disorders
2. To diagnose abnormalities in a fertilised egg before it is implanted in the mother's uterus
3. Tay-Sachs disease, haemophilia, Cystic fibrosis, fragile X syndrome, etc.

Q: What are the ways of screening Down syndrome?
Ans: There are three basic ways to screen:
1. *First trimester biochemical screening*: Assay of pregnancy-associated plasma protein A (PAPP-A) and hCG
2. *Second trimester biochemical screening*: The assay of maternal serum alpha-fetoprotein (MSAFP), hCG, oestriol, and inhibin.
3. Ultrasound for measuring nuchal translucency (NT) is another test for screening.
As per the guidelines by the department of Healtth (2010), first trimester combined screening (including a combination of NT and the first trimester biochemistry screening has now become the standard test for screening.

Q: Which tests are included in Triple test?
Ans: It involves with assay of AFP, free β-hCG, and oestriol.

Q: Which is the most commonly associated translocation in Down's syndrome?
Ans: Most commonly associated translocation is these cases are t (14; 21).

Q: What is the risk of Down's syndrome at age of 35 years?
Ans: 1 in 350

Q: Define spina bifida.

Ans: Congenital defect of the spine, which results from the failure of closure of the neural tube at 3–4 gestational weeks. In cases where the meninges protrude through this defect, it is called a meningocoele, and if neural tissues are also involved, it is known as a myelomeningocoele.

Q: What are the ultrasound findings in case of neural tube defects?
Ans: Ultrasound examination: 1. May show the "lemon sign", in which the foetal frontal bones are distorted
2. May also show the "banana sign" in which the shape of the cerebellum is altered

Q: At what gestational age is the routine ultrasound examination for assessment of congenital anomalies is recommended?
Ans: A routine ultrasound examination for assessment of congenital anomalies is recommended at 18–20^{+6} weeks of gestation.

Q: At what gestational age echogenic bowel is evident on ultrasound?
Ans: Echogenic bowel is evident in the form of "bright bowel" on ultrasound scan at 20 weeks.

Q: Name the condition associated with echogenic bowel.
Ans: Ecogenic bowel is a soft marker for down syndrome. Intra-amniotic haemorrhage with subsequent swallowing of blood products, cystic fibrosis, IUGR and intrauterine CMV infection are other causes for ecogenic bowel. VACTERL, another rare condition (1 in 6,000 births), may be associated with echogenic bowel. In these cases, baby has at least three of the following: Vertebral defects, Anal atresia, Cardiac abnormality, Tracheo-Esophageal fistula, Renal abnormalities, and Limb defects.

Q: What are the indications for administration of epidural anaesthesia?
Ans: 1. Provision of pain relief during first and second stages of labour
2. Facilitation of patient cooperation during labour and delivery
3. Provision of anaesthesia for episiotomy, forceps delivery, or extension for caesarean delivery

ONE-LINER QUESTIONS

Q: What is the site of insertion of epidural needle?
Ans: The epidural needle is inserted in the epidural space between the vertebra L3 and L4.

Q: How is epidural space identified at the time of needle insertion?
Ans: Epidural space can be identified by loss of resistance at the time of needle insertion.

Q: What are complications of epidural anaesthesia?
Ans: 1. Hypotension: due to pooling of blood in the periphery.
2. Increased incidence of malpositions
3. Risk of bleeding from the venous sinuses and haematoma formation

Q: What are the complications associated with caesarean deliveries performed under regional anaesthesia?
Ans: 1. Delayed respiratory depression with hydrophilic opioids
2. Venous air embolism
3. Evidence of myocardial ischaemia on the electrocardiograph
4. Postural headache

Q: What are the foetal side effects caused by pethidine analgesia in labour?
Ans: 1. Loss of beat-to-beat variability
2. Depression of the Apgar scores
3. Respiratory depression

Q: What is the time taken by pethidine analgesia to become apparent after administration?
Ans: The analgesic effects of pethidine becomes apparent after 10–15 minutes of administration

Q: What are constituents of Entonox? What are its uses?
Ans: Entonox is a gaseous mixture of nitrous oxide and oxygen. It is used for provision of analgesia during labour.

Q: What heart rate is considered normal in case of normal labour?

Ans: Heart rate of 110–160 beats per minute is normal.

Q: What are the causes of delay in the second stage of labour?
Ans: 1. The lack of expulsive sensation in the presence of an adequately working epidural
2. Maternal exhaustion

Q: What are causes of high/floating foetal head?
Ans: 1. Placenta praevia
2. Fibroid in the lower uterine segment
3. Pre-term infant

Q: What are the parameters plotted on the partogram?
Ans: Cervical dilatation and descent of the foetal presenting part at regular intervals; strength and frequency of contractions; maternal pulse, BP, and temperature; foetal heart rate; station of the presenting part; drugs and fluids administered; colour of liquor; interventions such as ARM, scalp pH measurement, etc.

Q: What are the foetal abnormalities which cause abnormal progress of labour?
Ans: 1. Abnormalities in foetal size (e.g. foetal macrosomia, with foetal weight >4,000 g)
2. Abnormalities in foetal presentation (e.g. brow, shoulder, face, etc.)
3. Abnormalities in foetal position (e.g. occiput posterior, occiput transverse, etc.)
4. Abnormalities in foetal attitude (extension, asynclitism, etc.)
5. Foetal congenital abnormalities (anencephaly, foetal ascites, foetal tumours, etc.).

Q: What are the characteristics of meconium in cystic fibrosis?
Ans: In cystic fibrosis, the meconium is thicker and collects in the ileum. This can present on the 20-week scan as bright echoes—"echogenic" or "bright" bowel. It may be shown as meconium ileus, characterised by failure to pass meconium, abdominal distension, and vomiting.

Q: What is the presentation of foetus in breech presentation?

ONE-LINER QUESTIONS

Ans: In Breech presentation, foetus lies longitudinally with the buttocks presenting in the lower pole of the uterus.

Q: Define cord prolapse (as defined by RCOG).
Ans: Descent of the umbilical cord through the cervix alongside the presenting part (occult presentation) or past it (overt presentation) in the presence of ruptured membranes

Q: Why classical caesarean delivery is still done occasionally?
Ans: This may be done in cases where lower segment may not be easily accessible due to fibroids; may be covered in enormous varicosities due to an anterior placenta praevia; or in presence of carcinoma cervix.

Q: Which incision is commonly used in caesarean section nowadays?
Ans: Pfannenstiel incision is commonly used.

Q: What are the factors that predispose to the formation of thrombus?
Ans: Endothelial injury, blood stasis, and hypercoagulability of blood

Q: What is the clinical presentation in cases of DVT?
Ans: 1. Pain in the calf muscles, oedema of legs
2. Rise in the skin temperature
3. Difference in the circumference between the affected and the normal leg may be more than 2 cm
4. Homan's sign is positive

Q: Define postpartum haemorrhage (according to WHO).
Ans: Excessive blood loss per vaginum (>500 mL in case of normal vaginal delivery or >1,000 mL following a caesarean section) from the time period extending within 24 hours of delivery and lasting until the end of the puerperium.

Q: What amount of blood loss occurs in primary PPH?
Ans: Blood loss is estimated to be greater than 500 mL, occurring from the genital tract, within 24 hours of delivery.

Q: What is secondary PPH?
Ans: Abnormal bleeding from the genital tract, which occurs 24 hours after delivery until 6 weeks post-partum.

Q: What are the characteristics of colostrum?
Ans: 1. Secretion of colostrum (a deep, lemon-yellow liquid) occurs from the breasts following delivery.
2. It contains high amounts of antibodies that help in protecting the newborn.
3. Colostrum contains high quantity of immunoglobulin A.
4. Colostrum is secreted for approximately the first 2 days post-partum

Q: Define mastitis.
Ans: 1. Defined as the parenchymatous infection of the mammary glands
2. Associated with milk stasis, nipple trauma, and poor nursing technique

Q: What is the mean red cell volume in a normal neonate?
Ans: Greater than 100 fl

Q: Name the various reflexes present in a newborn baby at birth.
Ans: 1. The stepping reflex
2. The Moro or startle reflex
3. Walking or stepping
4. Tonic neck reflex
5. The palmar and plantar grasp

Q: What does an APGAR score of 7 to 10 indicates?
Ans: Score between 7 and 10 indicates that the newborn is in good health
Score lower than 7 indicates that the baby requires some kind of medical attention

Q: Exomphalos can occur in association with which chromosomal abnormalities ?
Ans: T13 or T18

ONE-LINER QUESTIONS

Q: What are the causes of neonatal jaundice?
Ans: 1. Causes related to increased haemolysis: Spherocytosis and elliptocytosis, in which RBCs may be easily haemolysed.
2. Excessive load of blood may result in formation of excessive amounts of bilirubin, which the neonate may be unable to deal with.
3. A number of drugs such as sulphonamides, diazepam, etc. increase the risk for NJ.

Q: Which is the most commonly used form of therapy in neonatal jaundice?
Ans: Phototherapy

ONE-LINER QUESTIONS
Chapter 13
Gynaecology

Q: Administration of which antiemetic drug will result in development of movement disorder or neurological side effect?
Ans: Metoclopramide

Q: A bicornuate uterus is the result of failure of which embryonic structure to correctly fuse?
Ans: Paramesonephric ducts (Müllerian ducts)

Q: Which is the most specific enzyme indicator for myocardial infarction?
Ans: Troponin I

Q: Which is the most specific enzyme indicator for re-infarction?
Ans: Creatine kinase-MB

Q: What is the method of origin of bicornuate uterus?
Ans: Failure of fusion of paramesonephric duct

Q: Which injury can happen to a multiparous woman with descent of uterus (prolapsed)?
Ans: Cardinal/uterosacral ligaments

Q: The thick white vaginal discharge is characteristic of which infection?
Ans: *Candida*

Q: Which is the most common microorganism that causes UTI in postoperative patients with catheter?
Ans: *Pseudomonas*

Q: Uterus didephus results from failure of fusion of which structure?
Ans: Paramesonephric ducts

Q: Which is the main supporting ligament of uterus?
Ans: Cardinal ligament

Q: What is the most likely cause when patient is seen after hysterectomy with haemoglobin (Hb) 6.2 g/dL, haematocrit 29%, blood pressure 80/90 mm Hg, and pulse 109 bpm?
Ans: Internal bleeding

Q: Which enzyme is inhibited by finasteride?
Ans: 5-α reductase

Q: What is the most appropriate first-line pharmaceutical treatment for patient with no abnormalities on ultrasound scan and history of heavy regular periods?
Ans: Insertion of a LNG-IUS

Q: What is the probability of sarcomatous change occurring in fibroid?
Ans: 0.1%

Q: What is the main mechanism of action of the copper-IUD?
Ans: Inhibition of fertilization

Q: What percentage of women with over active bladder has urinary incontinence?
Ans: 1:3

Q: What can be the possible cause if the patient is presented with heavy vaginal discharge but no itching and have pH 6?
Ans: Bacterial vaginosis

Q: How many sperms are produced per 24 hours?
Ans: 30 million

Q: What is the most likely causative organism in case of fishy smelling vaginal odour with presence of clue cells in the smear?
Ans: *Gardnerella vaginalis*

ONE-LINER QUESTIONS

Q: Which ovarian tumour is most prone to undergo torsion during pregnancy?
Ans: Dermoid cyst

Q: Red degeneration of uterine fibroid during pregnancy is due to which pathological process?
Ans: Ischemia

Q: What is the description of *Neisseria gonorrhoeae*?
Ans: Gram-negative aerobic cocci

Q: What is the most common adverse effect experienced by women taking the progestogen-only pill?
Ans: Erratic bleeding

Q: What are the drugs used for pre-anaesthetic medication prior to gynaecological surgery?
Ans: Anxiolytic; antiemetic; H_2 blockers; anticholinergic; and analgesic drugs.

Q: Why is atropine used as pre-anaesthetic medication prior to gynaecological surgery?
Ans: Atropine is an anticholinergic. It is preferentially used to dry up secretions.

Q: Which is a commonly used skin cleanser and antiseptic?
Ans: Chlorhexidine

Q: Why is chlorhexidine a commonly used antiseptic solution prior to gynaecological surgery?
Ans: Because of its rapid action, broad-spectrum activity, and longer duration of action in comparison to the povidone-iodine solution.

Q: What is the mortality for peri-operative myocardial infarction?
Ans: The mortality for peri-operative myocardial infarction is approximately 40%.

Q: What is used as the specific markers of myocardial injury?

Ans: Presently, troponins are used as the specific markers of myocardial injury. Creatine kinase is an MB isoenzyme that peaks at 24–48 hours following myocardial infarction.

Q: What are the causes of hypertension frequently encountered amongst the operated patients in the immediate post-operative period?
Ans: Inadequate analgesic effect; hypercapnia; urinary retention; and diffusion hypoxia.

Q: What is the commonest cause of post-operative hypertension?
Ans: It is the inadequately controlled pain.

Q: What are the metabolic changes which occur in response to surgery in a normal person?
Ans: 1. The stress response and increased cortisol levels result in a relative hyperglycaemia, along with tachycardia.
2. Fluid retention and potassium loss
3. Rise in the metabolic rate

Q: What is the cause of pelvic and abdominal wound infection in the majority of cases?
Ans: The bacteria found amongst the endogenous microflora of the lower genital tract.

Q: What are the risk factors which predispose for development of wound infection?
Ans: Poor haemostasis; diabetes; rough handling of tissue; and tissue hypoxia.

Q: What is the difference between surgical wounds and non-surgical wounds?
Ans: Surgical wounds always have a source of infection, which can be drained surgically.

Q: Which is the commonest organism responsible for chronic osteomyelitis?
Ans: *Staphylococcus aureus*

ONE-LINER QUESTIONS

Q: Which are the commonest organisms to infect the surgical wound?
Ans: *Staphylococci* because they are common skin commensals.

Q: How is *Staphylococcus aureus* (MRSA) wound infection acquired and what are precautions to prevent this?
Ans: Methicillin-resistant *Staphylococcus aureus* (MRSA) wound infection is hospital-acquired. The risk of acquisition can be minimised by observing precautions like handwashing before wound inspection.

Q: Why surgical wounds become infected with opportunistic organisms?
Ans: Because of the relatively immunocompromised state of the post-operative patient resulting in reduced inhibition of microbial growth.

Q: What is necrotising fasciitis and how is this caused?
Ans: A deep-seated aggressive infection of subcutaneous tissue and skin (commonly caused by group A *Streptococci*).

Q: Mention the commonest aerobic bacteria isolated from the intra-abdominal pus in descending order.
Ans: 1. *Escherichia coli*
2. *Enterococci*
3. *Proteus*
4. *Klebsiella* spp.

Q: Mention the commonest anaerobic bacteria in descending order.
Ans: 1. *Bacteroides*
2. *Clostridia*
3. *Peptostreptococci*

Q: Which anaerobes are commonly found in breast abscesses?
Ans: *Actinomyces* and *Bacillus*

Q: What are the resultants of defective wound healing?
Ans: 1. Superficial wound disruption

2. Incisional hernias
3. Cicatrisation
4. Wound dehiscence

Q: Are hypertrophic scarring and keloid formation results of defective wound healing?
Ans: No. They are not the results of defective wound healing.

Q: What are features of keloid scarring?
Ans: 1. Keloid scars are characterised by smooth hard nodules caused by excessive collagen production.
2. Commoner in people of Afro-Caribbean origin.
3. Associated with skin trauma, infection, and surgery.
4. If keloid scarring is treated with surgical removal then it must be followed by steroid injection or superficial radiotherapy.
5. Primary wound closure is a risk factor.
6. Methods of treatment include triamcinolone injection and compression with silica gels.

Q: By which factors the metabolic response to trauma is mediated?
Ans: By both endocrine and paracrine factors.

Q: What results in thirst?
Ans: Increased secretion of ADH results in thirst. Thirst also occurs due to the stimulation of the thirst receptors.

Q: What are the side effects of total parenteral nutrition (TPN)?
Ans: Catheter-related sepsis and metabolic abnormalities resulting from the administered nutrients.

Q: What is the composition and osmolarity of TPN?
Ans: TPN is hyperosmolar. It typically contains about 250 g glucose and 14–16 g of L-amino acids.

Q: With which metabolic disturbances TPN is associated with?
Ans: Deficiency of fatty acids; hyperchloraemic metabolic acidosis; hypercarbia; hyperglycaemia; hypovolaemia; and hypoglycaemia.

Q: What is the strategy on which contraceptive methods are based?

Ans: Three general strategies: prevention of ovulation; prevention of fertilization, or prevention of implantation.

Q: What is the failure rate of barrier contraceptives?
Ans: Failure rate of 9–30 per 100 women years of use.

Q: What are the commonly used barrier methods of contraception?
Ans: Male condom, female condom, diaphragm, cervical cap, vaginal sponge, and spermicides.

Q: What is the failure rate of condom?
Ans: Failure rates of 10–15 per 100 woman years are quoted for the condom.

Q: What is the recommendation of The Family Planning Association (FPA, 2014), UK regarding use of spermicides with latex condoms?
Ans: It advises that spermicides should not be used with latex condoms and that spermicides do not offer additional contraceptive efficacy when used in conjunction with latex condoms.

Q: What is the material used in female condom?
Ans: Strong, soft, transparent polyurethane sheath

Q: What are contraindications of use of diaphragm?
Ans: Man or woman has allergy to rubber, latex, or spermicide.
2. Woman has frequent urinary tract or bladder infections.
3. Woman has anatomical abnormalities.

Q: How much hours of protection is provided by cervical cap?
Ans: 48 hours.

Q: What are the complications associated with use of cervical cap?
Ans: Toxic shock syndrome, unpleasant odour, discomfort and awareness of the cap during coitus, and accidental dislodgment.

Q: What are the basic components of spermicides?

Ans: Surfactants (Nonoxynol-9, Octoxynol-9, Menfegol) and the base (carrier) agent (e.g. foams, jellies, creams, foaming tablet, melting suppositories, aerosols, soluble films, or vaginal suppositories).

Q: What are the various formulations of progestogen-only contraceptive methods?
Ans: 1. Progestogen-only pill (POP) or minipill
2. Sub-dermal contraceptive implants (Norplant I, II, and Implanon)
3. Progestogen-only injectables (POI), e.g. depot medroxyprogesterone acetate (DMPA)
4. Intrauterine system (Mirena and progestasert).

Q: What is composition of the progestogen-only pill?
Ans: 50 μg of norethisterone or 75 μg of norgestrel or 30 μg of levonorgestrel.

Q: What is mechanism of action of oral progestogens?
Ans: 1. They act by causing increased viscosity of cervical mucus and endometrial changes.
2. Progestogens induce a premature secretory change in the endometrium, thereby making it unfavourable for implantation.
3. The POP decreases tubal motility, hence its association with tubal ectopic pregnancy.

Q: Mention the cases in which POPs are prescribed?
Ans: 1. Hypertension, superficial thrombophlebitis, history of thromboembolism, biliary tract disease, thyroid disease, epilepsy, diabetes without vascular disease, etc.
2. Following delivery
3. Lactation

Q: Why minipills are recommended over COCPs in women who are breastfeeding?
Ans: Because they do not affect milk production.

Q: Which are the first-generation, second-generation, and third-generation progestins?
Ans: First-generation: Norethindrone, norethindrone acetate, and ethynodiol diacetate

ONE-LINER QUESTIONS

Second-generation progestins: Levonorgestrel
Third-generation progestins: Desogestrel, gestodene, and norgestimate.

Q: What is the method of administration of injectable progestogens?
Ans: Deep intramuscular injections are given into the muscles of the arms or buttocks.

Q: What are the two main types of POIs?
Ans: DMPA and norethisterone enanthate (NETEN).

Q: How many times in a year injectable progestogens are given?
Ans: Four times a year (every 11–13 weeks).

Q: Why injection site should not be massaged after injectable progestogens are injected?
Ans: The injection site should not be massaged afterwards, because this may accelerate absorption of the drug.

Q: What is the failure rate of injectable contraceptives?
Ans: 0.1–0.4%.

Q: What is composition of Depo-provera?
Ans: It contains 150 mg medroxyprogesterone in an aqueous microcrystalline suspension.

Q: Mention names of copper carrying devices.
Ans: Copper T 200, copper 7, multiload, copper 250, copper T 380, copper T 220, and nova T.

Q: What is effective life of copper carrying devices?
Ans: From 3 to 5 years

Q: Name intrauterine contraceptive devices containing progestogen.
Ans: Progestasert, levonova, and Mirena.

Q: What is the amount of levonorgestrel in Mirena?

Ans: Mirena contains 52 mg of levonorgestrel (which is released at the rate of 20 µg/day).

Q: What is effective life of Mirena?
Ans: 5 years.

Q: What is another name for Mirena?
Ans: Levonorgestrel-intrauterine system (LNGIUS)

Q: What are commonest side effects of intrauterine devices in the first month after insertion?
Ans: Irregular menstrual bleeding, spotting, menorrhagia, etc.

Q: When does uterine perforation occurs after IUD insertion?
Ans: This may occur either at the time of insertion or at a later stage (due to the embedment of the device into the myometrium and its subsequent migration into the intra-abdominal cavity).

Q: What is the pregnancy rate in contraception from intrauterine contraceptive devices?
Ans: Pregnancy rate is 0.1–1 per 100 women years.

Q: How many types of COCPs formulations are available?
Ans: Three types: monophasic pills, biphasic pills, and triphasic pills.

Q: What are the adverse effects related to the use of COCPs which need to be reported?
Ans: 1. A—Abdominal pain (severe)
2. C—Chest pain (severe), cough, shortness of breath or sharp pain upon breathing
3. H—Headache (severe), dizziness, weakness, or numbness (especially one-sided)
4. E—Eye problems (complete loss of or blurring of vision)
5. S—Severe leg pain (calf or thigh).

Q: What is morning-after pill?
Ans: Morning-after pill/emergency contraception (EC)/post-coital contraception is a method of contraception. This is used after intercourse and before the potential time of implantation.

ONE-LINER QUESTIONS

Q: What is Yuzpe method of contraception?
Ans: This method comprises of the oral administration of two doses of 100 µg ethinyl estradiol and 500 µg levonorgestrel taken 12 hours apart.

Q: Which progesterone receptor modulator got licensed for EC in 2009?
Ans: Ulipristal

Q: What are the indications for the use of EC?
Ans: 1. Failure to use a contraceptive method
2. Condom breakage or leakage
3. Dislodgement of a diaphragm or a cervical cap
4. Two or more missed birth control pills
5. Depo-provera injection is late by 1 week or more
7. Sexual assault when the woman is not using reliable contraception.

Q: Which contraceptive method legal status as emergency contraception in the UK changed from a prescription only medicine to a pharmacy medicine in January 2001?
Ans: LNG

Q: Which forms of LNG are available in market?
Ans: It is available as "Levonelle One Step" and "Levonelle 1500" and comprise of one 1500 microgram tablet to be taken within 72 hours of an unprotected intercourse. The previously available 0.75 mg tablets were "Levonelle 2".

Q: What are the common side effects of hormonal EC?
Ans: Gastrointestinal and mainly include nausea, vomiting, dizziness, and fatigue.

Q: What are the possible complications of post-coital IUD insertion?
Ans: Pelvic pain, abnormal bleeding, pelvic infection, perforation, and expulsion.

Q: What is primary and secondary amenorrhoea?
Ans: *Primary amenorrhoea*: Woman has never experienced menstrual cycles
1. Absence of menses by age of 14 years with the absence of growth or development of secondary sexual characteristics
2. Absence of menses by the age of 16 years with normal development of secondary sexual characteristics.

Secondary amenorrhoea: Woman had experienced menstrual bleeding previously before experiencing cessation for at least 6 months. Cessation of menstruation for more than 6 months, but not attributable to pregnancy or the menopause.

Q: Define cryptomenorrhoea.
Ans: Cryptomenorrhoea means "hidden menstruation". This implies that though menstruation occurs, the menstrual blood remains concealed.

Q: What are the conditions in which cryptomenorrhoea can occur?
Ans: Imperforate hymen; cervical stenosis after cone biopsy or Manchester repair or rarely due to the congenital absence of the vagina.

Q: What is the usual presentation of cryptomenorrhoea?
Ans: The usual presentation is a pubertal girl with primary amenorrhoea, recurrent abdominal pain, and an imperforate hymen.

Q: How is haematocolpos and haematometra caused?
Ans: The accumulation of menstrual blood within the vagina and the uterus results in the development of haematocolpos and haematometra, respectively.

Q: Define infertility.
Ans: The inability to conceive even after trying with unprotected intercourse for a period of 1 year for couples in which the woman is less than 35 years and 6 months of trying for couples in which the woman is more than 35 years of age.

Q: Which vitamin prevents sperm DNA damage?

ONE-LINER QUESTIONS

Ans: Vitamin E can help counter oxidative stress, which is associated with sperm DNA damage.

Q: Which drug is used in the patients with ejaculatory sexual dysfunction?
Ans: Phosphodiesterase Type 5 inhibitors (e.g. sildenafil).

Q: Which is an effective therapy for impotence and is generally used following failure of oral phosphodiesterase inhibitors?
Ans: Caverject (intracavernosal alprostadil).

Q: In which cases squeeze technique is used?
Ans: The squeeze technique (where the penile shaft is firmly squeezed during intercourse) can help in the treatment of premature ejaculation.

Q: Which drug is used for treatment of premature ejaculation?
Ans: Fluoxetine can be a useful treatment for premature ejaculation.

Q: Name the procedures included in assisted reproductive techniques.
Ans: Sperm washing/capacitation, intrauterine insemination, gamete intra-fallopian transfer, in vitro fertilisation (IVF), and micromanipulation [intra-cytoplasmic sperm injection (ICSI)].

Q: Which technique has successful outcomes in men with Klinefelter's syndrome?
Ans: ICSI.

Q: What are the primary values that are evaluated at the time of semen analysis?
Ans: Volume of the ejaculate, sperm motility, total sperm concentration, sperm morphology, motility, and viability.

Q: What are the causes of female infertility?
Ans: 1. Previous ectopic pregnancy
2. Previous pelvic infection
3. Cystic fibrosis (in a male)

4. Reversal of vasectomy (in a male)

Q: What is teratozoospermia?
Ans: Excess of abnormally formed spermatozoa

Q: What is azoospermia?
Ans: No spermatozoa in the semen

Q: Which are the criteria [according to the American Society of Reproductive Medicine (ASRM) and the European Society of Human Reproduction and Embryology (ESHRE) joint consensus meeting in November 2003] for the diagnosis of PCOS?
Ans: Diagnosis of PCOS should be made, when two of the following three criteria are met:
1. Infrequent or absent ovulation
2. Clinical or biochemical features of hyperandrogenism, such as excessive hair growth, acne, raised LH and raised androgen levels
3. Morphologically, there is bilateral ovarian enlargement, thickened ovarian capsule, multiple follicular cysts

Q: What are the features of polycystic ovarian syndrome?
Ans: Infrequent or absent ovulation; obesity; hirsutism; oligomenorrhea; the risk of endometrial hyperplasia and carcinoma may be increased; and miscarriage and infertility.

Q: What are the features of polycystic ovarian morphology on ultrasound scan?
Ans: 1. Greater than 12 follicles measuring between 2 mm and 9 mm in diameter, located peripherally, resulting in a pearl necklace appearance
2. Increased echogenicity of ovarian stroma and/or ovarian volume greater than 10 mL

Q: What is the treatment of choice in patients with PCOS in ovulation induction?
Ans: Clomiphene citrate

Q: Which drug is the first line of management in cases of clomiphene citrate-resistant women with PCOS?

ONE-LINER QUESTIONS

Ans: Metformin.

Q: In which patients ovarian hyperstimulation syndrome occurs?
Ans: It occurs in patients undergoing ovulation induction with clomiphene or human menopausal gonadotropin (hMG) or controlled ovarian hyperstimulation for assisted reproductive technologies.

Q: In presence of which conditions, ovarian hyperstimulation is more common?
Ans: 1. When there are many follicles (say more than 15)
2. When the plasma oestrogen level has exceeded 2,500 pg/mL on the day of hCG administration
3. Where pregnancy has occurred.

Q: What are the characteristics of Asherman's syndrome?
Ans: 1. Development of intrauterine adhesions (occurring in women who have had endometrial trauma associated with vigorous curettage, especially following abortion or delivery).
2. These adhesions may cause amenorrhoea, repeated miscarriages, infertility, and ectopic pregnancy.
3. Diagnosis is done by tests like hysteroscopy and transvaginal ultrasound examination.
3. Treatment involves hysteroscopic surgery to cut and remove the adhesions or scar tissue.

Q: Which is the most important cause of fallopian tube obstruction?
Ans: Pelvic inflammatory disease (PID)

Q: What are test for tubal patency?
Ans: 1. The injection of a radio-opaque aqueous solution through the cervix under radiographic control.
2. Laparoscopic examination of the uterus and fallopian tubes: Method of choice for investigating tubal patency.

Q: What are the causes of dyspareunia?
Ans: Deep retroverted uterus with prolapsed ovaries (the "ovarian entrapment" syndrome); superficial vulvovaginitis (especially

infection by *Trichomonas* or *Candida*); vaginal cysts; infection of Bartholin's gland; post-menopausal shrinkage; endometriosis/adenomyosis; chronic pelvic infection; pelvic tumours including ectopic pregnancy; and thick hymen (rarely).

Q: What are the types of urogenital fistulas?
Ans: 1. Urethrovaginal
2. Vesical fistula [vesicovaginal fistula (VVF) or vesicocervical]
3. Ureterovaginal
4. Rectovaginal

Q: What is vesicovaginal fistula?
Ans: An abnormal fistulous tract extending between the bladder and the vagina that allows the continuous involuntary discharge of urine into the vaginal vault.

Q: What is the principle of the surgery of vesicovaginal fistulae?
Ans: Most of the VVF can be closed by surgery via the vaginal route. The principle of the surgery is to separate the bladder mucosa from the vaginal skin. The mucosa is then carefully closed in one or two layers, without tension, using polyglycolic acid sutures.

Q: Define uterine prolapse.
Ans: It is descent or herniation of the uterus into or beyond the vagina.
Cystocoele and urethrocoele: Due to weakness of the anterior compartment
Descent of uterine vault or uterine prolapse and enterocoele: Due to weakness of the middle compartment
Rectocoele: Due to the weakness of the posterior compartment

Q: What are the symptoms of pelvic prolapse?
Ans: 1. Vaginal discomfort, dragging and the sensation of "something coming down" the vagina, sensation of lump in the vagina, a feeling of pelvic insecurity, and low backache.
2. Backache
3. Urinary symptoms, such as difficulty in passing urine and recurrent UTIs
4. Difficulty in passing stool.

ONE-LINER QUESTIONS

5. Blood stained vaginal discharge
6. Dyspareunia

Q: Which are the most important ligaments supporting the uterus?
Ans: Transverse cervical or cardinal ligaments that attach the cervix and vaginal vault to the sidewalls of the pelvis

Q: Which is the most important muscle of the pelvic floor?
Ans: The levator ani muscle

Q: What are the divisions of levator ani muscle?
Ans: Three main divisions: (1) pubococcygeus, (2) iliococcygeus, and (3) ischiococcygeus.

Q: What is the shape of perineal body?
Ans: Pyramid-shaped fibro-muscular structure lying at the centre of perineum (midpoint between the vagina and the anus)

Q: Which muscles are attached to perineal body?
Ans: Eight muscles of the pelvic floor: superficial and deep transverse perineal muscles; levator ani muscles of both the sides; bulbocavernosus anteriorly, and the external anal sphincter posteriorly

Q: What is ring pessary?
Ans: Pessaries are a non-surgical method for supporting the uterine and vaginal structures

Q: What are the indications of Manchester operation?
Ans: 1. Childbearing function is not required.
2. Malignancy of the endometrium has been ruled out by performing a dilatation and curettage.
3. Absence of UTI
4. Presence of a small cystocoele with only first- or second-degree prolapse
5. Absence of an enterocoele

Q: What is stress incontinence?

Ans: SUI is involuntary leakage of urine during conditions, which causes an increase in intra-abdominal pressure (exertion, sneezing, coughing, or exercise) causing the intra-vesical pressure to rise higher than that which the urethral closure mechanisms can withstand (in the absence of detrusor contractions).

Q: Which is the fundamental test of bladder function and measures changes in bladder pressure with changes in bladder volume?
Ans: Cystometry

Q: What are the procedures available for urinary incontinence?
Ans: Transvaginal urethropexies/needle suspension procedures/Pereyra's procedure; retropubic bladder neck suspension procedures or colposuspension; sub-urethral sling procedures, and periurethral injections.

Q: What is voiding pressure in urodynamic study in normal adult female?
Ans: 45–70 cm H_2O

Q: What is bladder capacity in urodynamic study in normal adult female?
Ans: 400–600 mL

Q: Which methods are used for stress incontinence resulting from intrinsic sphincteric damage or weakness?
Ans: Sub-urethral sling procedures and peri-urethral injections

Q: Name the bulking agents used in peri-urethral injections?
Ans: Collagen; carbon-coated zirconium; ethylene vinyl alcohol; polydimethylsiloxane; polytetrafluoroethylene; and glutaraldehyde cross-linked bovine collagen (contigen).

Q: How is urge incontinence caused?
Ans: By uninhibited contractions of the detrusor muscle

Q: What is management of urge incontinence?

ONE-LINER QUESTIONS

Ans: 1. *First-line treatment*: Behavioural therapies such as bladder training and bladder drill help in establishing or re-establishing cortical control over a hyperactive micturition reflex
2. *Second-line treatment*: Medical treatment—anti-cholinergic drugs oxybutynin (Ditropan) or imipramine (Tofranil)
3. *Third-line treatment*: Surgical procedures (rarely used)

Q: Which is the main smooth muscle relaxant used in the case of urge incontinence?
Ans: Oxybutynin (in the dosage of 5 mg, 2–4 times per day)

Q: Which is the most appropriate technique for patients with detrusor hyperreflexia and functional obstruction?
Ans: Intermittent catheterisation

Q: What is the type of hair in hirsutism?
Ans: In cases of hirsutism, there are excessive hair called "terminal" hair (which are coarse and pigmented).

Q: How is hirsutism scored?
Ans: By using the modified Ferriman-Gallwey system. A score of greater than 8 is considered as diagnostic.

Q: Which is the major cause of hirsuitism?
Ans: Polycystic ovary syndrome (up to 80% of all cases)

Q: What is the composition of *Yasmin®*?
Ans: Trade name of an oral contraceptive pill comprising 30 µg ethinyl oestradiol and 3 mg drospirenone. Drospirenone is a derivative of spironolactone and has similar anti-androgenic properties.

Q: Which are the commonest ovarian tumours in pregnancy?
Ans: Dermoid cysts of the ovary (benign cystic teratomas)

Q: What is normal position of uterus?
Ans: Anteversion and anteflexion

Q: What is the position of uterus in retroversion?
Ans: Uterine body is displaced backwards at the utero-cervical junction

Q: Which conditions are related to fixed retroversion?
Ans: It could be related to conditions such as PID (salpingo-oophoritis), pelvic tumours, chocolate cysts of the ovary, and pelvic endometriosis.

Q: Which pessary is used in cases of symptomatic mobile retroversion?
Ans: Hodge pessary

Q: Which is the most commonly used surgical option in fixed retroversion?
Ans: Modified Gillam's ventrosuspension

Q: What are the symptoms of fibroids?
Ans: Anaemia (due to excessive bleeding), bleeding, pressure symptoms (e.g. urinary symptoms, low backache, rectal tenesmus, and constipation), and less commonly pain. The pattern of bleeding is usually excessive or prolonged menses (menorrhagia).

Q: What are the options of surgical treatment of uterine fibroids?
Ans: Endoscopic myomectomy, abdominal hysterectomy, abdominal myomectomy, vaginal myomectomy, and vaginal hysterectomy.

Q: What is uterine artery embolization?
Ans: UAE is a non-hysterectomy surgical technique that helps in reducing the size of the uterine fibroids by shrinking them, without actually removing them.

Q: What is the composition of embolising agent in uterine artery embolization?
Ans: An embolising agent consists of gelatin microspheres (trisacryl gelatin) or polyvinyl alcohol.

Q: What are degenerative changes taking place in the fibroids?
Ans: 1. Shrinkage of the fibroid

ONE-LINER QUESTIONS

2. Hyaline degeneration
3. Calcification of the fibroid
4. Myxomatous/cystic degeneration
5. Red/carneous degeneration of uterine fibroid

Q: What is difference between red degeneration of fibroids and placental abruption?
Ans: *Red degeneration*: There is no bleeding; the area of pain and tenderness is localised to the fibroid; the rest of the uterus is soft; and the foetal heart rate is normal.
Placental abruption: Bleeding is usually present. There may be an evidence of shock. The uterus is "woody" hard and tender all over; foetal parts are difficult to feel and localise; and foetal heart activity cannot be usually detected.

Q: Define primary and secondary dysmenorrhea.
Ans: *Primary dysmenorrhea*: Spasmodic or the 1st day pain; absence of underlying medical disease/pathology.
Secondary dysmenorrhea: Congestive type; associated with an underlying medical disease/pathology.

Q: What results in bicornuate uterus?
Ans: It occurs due to abnormality of the fusion process in the upper parts of Mullerian ducts. There is a single cervical canal in the lower part, but the upper part is bifurcated, having two horns.

Q: Which is the commonest type of uterine malformation?
Ans: Uterus malformation resulting due to the incomplete fusion of the Müllerian ducts or paramesonephric ducts.

Q: What are the characteristics of uterus didelphys?
Ans: Double vagina; double cervix; and entirely double uterus, that is, two single-horned uteruses

Q: What are the various theories behind the origin of endometriosis?
Ans: 1. Theory of coelomic metaplasia: Peritoneal epithelium can get "transformed" into endometrial tissue under the influence of some unknown stimulus.

2. Metastatic deposition of endometrial tissues at ectopic sites can occur via lymphatic and vascular routes.
3. Immunological defects and genetic factors.

Q: What are the features of endometriosis?
Ans: Dysmenorrhoea; deep dyspareunia; chocolate cysts of the ovaries (due to collection of old blood/clotted blood), and fixed retroversion of the uterus. Rarely, bowel symptoms may be present.

Q: Which bacteria are present in normal vaginal epithelium?
Ans: The normal vaginal epithelium contains numerous bacteria called *L. acidophilus*.

Q: What are Amsel's diagnostic criteria for bacterial vaginosis?
Ans: 1. Thin, homogeneous discharge
2. Positive "Whiff test"
3. Presence of "clue cells" on microscopic examination
4. Vaginal pH greater than 4.5

Q: What is the dose of metronidazole in bacterial vaginosis?
Ans: A 7-day course of oral metronidazole, 400 mg TDS or vaginal metronidazole gel (metrogel) is an effective treatment.

Q: Which is the treatment of choice in pregnancy for BV?
Ans: Clindamycin. This has been shown to reduce the risk of pre-term delivery.

Q: What is the drug of choice for treatment of candidal infections? What is its dose?
Ans: Fluconazole. Fluconazole (Diflucan) is available to the public in a 150 mg single-dose preparation.

Q: What is the mode of spreading of gonorrhoea?
Ans: It spreads through contact with the penis, vagina, mouth, or anus. It can also spread from mother to baby at the time of delivery.

Q: What are the causes for painful genital ulcers?
Ans: Herpes simplex/zoster and genital herpes; Behcet's disease; Reiter's syndrome; chancroid; and gonococcal disease.

ONE-LINER QUESTIONS

Q: What is Fitz-Hugh-Curtis Syndrome?
Ans: This syndrome is related to peri-hepatic infection with formation of fine adhesions known as the "violin string" secondary to pelvic infection.

Q: What is the position of Bartholin's glands?
Ans: The Bartholin's glands are situated at the level of the introitus within the labia majora.

Q: How is cyst of Bartholin's glands treated?
Ans: Treatment is by "marsupialisation", in which the cyst is effectively de-roofed to allow drainage.

Q: What is the standard treatment in cases of genital warts? Can this be followed in pregnancy?
Ans: Podophyllin in spirit. It can be toxic in pregnancy; so, it is not to be used.

Q: What is the mode of transmission of genital herpes?
Ans: It spreads only by direct person-to-person contact. The virus enters through the mucous membrane of the genital tract via microscopic tears. From there, the virus travels to the nerve roots near the spinal cord and settles down permanently.

Q: What are symptoms of genital herpes?
Ans: 1. Constitutional symptoms like fever, malaise, vulval paraesthesia, itching or tingling sensation on the vulva and vagina followed by redness of skin
2. Blisters and vesicles on the vulva, vagina, cervix, perianal area, or inner thigh (which ultimately develop into shallow and painful ulcers within a period of 2–6 weeks)
3. They are frequently accompanied by itching and mucoid vaginal discharge.
4. Swollen and tender lymph nodes may occur in the groin region.

Q: What is the Tzanck smear method?

Ans: 1. Rapid, fairly sensitive, and inexpensive method for diagnosing HSV infection
2. Smears are prepared from the base of the lesions and stained with 1% aqueous solution of toluidine blue "O" for 15 seconds.
3. Multi-nucleated giant cells with faceted nuclei and homogeneously stained "ground glass" chromatin (Tzanck cells) indicates positive smear.

: What are the complications of non-gonococcal urethritis (NGU)?
Ans: Salpingitis, peri-hepatitis, conjunctivitis, and sterility.

ONE-LINER QUESTIONS

CHAPTER 14
Endocrinology

Q: Insulin gets active by removing which part?
Ans: C-peptide

Q: What is the most common thyroid disease in a female in child bearing period?
Ans: Grave's disease

Q: Hormone replacement therapy reduces the risk of which cancer?
Ans: Colorectal cancer

Q: Which cell type secretes calcitonin?
Ans: Parafollicular cells (C-cells)

Q: Which drug is causing grey baby syndrome?
Ans: Chloramphenicol

Q: Which drug is causing Redman syndrome?
Ans: Vancomycin

Q: Which is the most common cause for osteoporosis?
Ans: Old age

Q: Which is the most important cause for insulin deficiency?
Ans: Diabetes ketoacidosis

Q: Vasopressin act on which part of the kidney for increasing water re-absorption?
Ans: Distal convoluted tubules and collecting duct

Q: Which is the soft haemorrhage ovarian tumour with Call-Exner bodies?
Ans: Granulosa cell tumour

Q: Which hormone is helpful in sodium absorption?
Ans: Aldosterone

Q: What is the percentage of free T4 in non-pregnant woman?
Ans: 1%

Q: Androgens are produced by which cells?
Ans: Theca cells

Q: What is prolactin inhibitor dopamine agonist?
Ans: Quinagolide

Q: Which type of tumour increase growth hormone secretion lead to acromegaly?
Ans: Adenoma

Q: What kind of cells produces parathyroid hormone (PTH)?
Ans: Chief cells

Q: What day of a regular 25-day menstrual cycle is a woman likely to ovulate?
Ans: 11

Q: What is the chemical structure of gonadotropin-releasing hormone (GnRH)?
Ans: Decapeptide

Q: What is the most potent and abundant form of oestrogen in postmenopausal women?
Ans: Oestrone

Q: Which hormone promotes cartilage mitosis in epiphyseal plate of long bones?
Ans: Growth hormone

Q: What inhibit glucagon release?
Ans: Increased fatty acid

Q: What is the most common cause of hyperprolactinemia?

ONE-LINER QUESTIONS

Ans: Primary hypothyroidism

Q: What is non-ergot dopamine agonist drug used to treat hyperprolactinemia?
Ans: Quinagolide

Q: How many days does it take from the resting follicle stage to ovulation?
Ans: 14 days

Q: Luteinising hormone peak precedes ovulation by how much time?
Ans: 10–12 hours

Q: Which in the best way describes the histological type of endometrium soon after ovulation?
Ans: Secretory endometrium

Q: Which eicosanoid mainly increases before menstruation?
Ans: Prostaglandin F2α

Q: What is the most common cause of secondary hyperparathyroidism?
Ans: Chronic renal failure

Q: What is the most common cause of delay in puberty in males?
Ans: Constitutional delay in growth

Q: Which hormone is secreted by the placenta and foetal adrenal gland and promotes maturation of the foetal lungs?
Ans: Cortisol

Q: What is the major oestrogen produced by the placenta during pregnancy?
Ans: Oestriol

Q: What is the most common inherited bleeding disorder?
Ans: Von Willebrand's disease

Q: Which chemical concentration increases before menstruation?
Ans: Prostaglandin F2α

Q: Which hormonal abnormality results in increased sweating during pregnancy?
Ans: Thyroid

Q: Which enzyme causes excretion of calcium?
Ans: Calcitonin

Q: Which is the earliest physical sign of puberty in females?
Ans: Thelarche

Q: What type of compound is thyroid releasing hormone (TRH)?
Ans: Protein

Q: What is the most common cause of Cushing's syndrome?
Ans: Iatrogenic steroid administration

Q: Human placental lactogen (hPL) is structurally MOST similar to which hormone?
Ans: Growth hormone

Q: What is the single best description for the histological appearance of the secretory endometrium?
Ans: Simple columnar epithelium with subnuclear vacuolation

Q: Androgen is secreted from which region of the adrenal gland?
Ans: Zona reticularis

Q: Which hormone prevents regression of corpus luteum?
Ans: Human chorionic gonadotrophin

Q: What happens to calcium and phosphate levels in a patient with primary hyperparathyroidism?
Ans: Increased calcium levels and reduced phosphate levels.

Q: Where is ADH synthesized?
Ans: Paraventricular nucleus of the hypothalamus

ONE-LINER QUESTIONS

Q: What is the most common cause of hyperthyroidism in young woman?
Ans: Grave's disease

Q: Which hormone causes rupture of graafian follicle and release of oestrogen and progesterone?
Ans: Luteinising hormone

Q: List various male hormones in the increasing order of potency.
Ans: Dihydrotestosterone (DHT) (most potent) >Testosterone >Androstenedione A2 >DHEA (least potent)

Q: Which organ anomaly occurs with the use of ACE inhibitor?
Ans: Kidney

Q: What type of glands are the endocrine glands?
Ans: ductless

Q: Other than endocrine glands, which other organs also produce hormones?
Ans: Gonads and other organs such as thymus, kidneys, heart, and placenta.

Q: On what factors placenta is dependent for steroidogenesis?
Ans: It depends upon the precursors derived from the foetal and partly from the maternal sources.

Q: What is the half-life of insulin? What is its advantage?
Ans: Half-life of insulin is between 5 hours and 10 hours. This short half-life allows an accurate control of the blood glucose levels.

Q: Why is half-life of thyroxine longer than that of triiodothyronine?
Ans: Because it is more highly protein-bound which appears to prolong its life.

Q: Which hormones show characteristic of diurnal variation?

Ans: It is characteristic of hormones such as cortisol, testosterone, and melatonin and to a lesser extent growth hormone (GH) (pulses).

Q: Name the hormones which are peptide in nature.
Ans: 1. *Short polypeptide chains and small proteins*: ADH, oxytocin, GH and prolactin, adrenocorticotrophic hormone (ACTH), parathormone, calcitonin, insulin, glucagon, somatostatin, pancreatic polypeptide, hCG, human chorionic somatomammotrophin, etc.
2. *Glycoprotein hormones*: Thyroid-stimulating hormone (TSH), luteinising hormone (LH), and follicle-stimulating hormone (FSH).

Q: What is the structure of steroid hormones?
Ans: These are synthesised from cholesterol and have the same basic 4-ring structure composed of 17 carbon atoms with different number of carbon atoms added in form of side chains. Three rings A, B, and C are composed of 6 carbon atoms, whereas the last ring (D) is composed of 5-carbon atoms.

Q: Name the hormones which are steroid in nature.
Ans: Oestrogens, androgens, mineralocorticoids, and glucocorticoids.

Q: Name the hormones which are amino acid in nature.
Ans: Thyroid hormones, catecholamines, and melatonin.

Q: Which hormones are derived from the amino acid tyrosine?
Ans: Thyroxine (T4), triiodothyronine (T3), adrenaline (epinephrine), noradrenaline (norepinephrine), and dopamine.

Q: Which hormones are derived from the amino acid tryptophan?
Ans: Melatonin

Q: What is sex hormone binding globulin (SHBG)?
Ans: SHBG is a β-globulin that transports androgens [e.g. testosterone, dihydrotestosterone (DHT), androstenedione and dehydroepiandrosterone] and oestradiol in plasma.

Q: Define hormone receptors.

ONE-LINER QUESTIONS

Ans: These are the large proteins present in the target cells. Each receptor is specific for one single hormone.

Q: Where are the receptors of protein hormones and adrenal medullary hormones (catecholamines) present?
Ans: Cell membrane

Q: Where are the receptors of steroid hormones present?
Ans: Nucleus

Q: What is the embryological origin of thalamus and the hypothalamus?
Ans: Develop from the lateral walls of the diencephalon

Q: Which gland lies within a bony depression in the sphenoid bone, the sella turcica?
Ans: The pituitary gland

Q: What is the embryological origin of pituitary gland?
Ans: 1. *Adenophysis*: Develops from Rathke's pouch, an upward evagination of the ectoderm of the pharyngeal roof.
2. *Neurohypophysis*: Develops from a neuroectodermal down growth from the floor of the third ventricle.

Q: Which hormones are secreted from the posterior lobe of the pituitary?
Ans: Oxytocin and vasopressin

Q: What is chromophobe adenoma?
Ans: It refers to the lack of uptake of staining within the pituitary tumour which means that the tumour is non-functioning.

Q: What is role of melatonin?
Ans: It has a role in the regulation of circadian rhythm (body's biological clock) and puberty.

Q: What is the location of genes for human GH?

Ans: These are localised in the q22-24 region of chromosome 17 and are closely related to human placental lactogen (hPL) genes.

Q: How does secretion of GH varies during pregnancy?
Ans: Secretion of GH during pregnancy is not increased; it may actually be reduced because of the increased level of hPL.

Q: Does impaired GH secretion in children cause delayed puberty?
Ans: Pituitary gonadotropins determine the time of onset of puberty. GH does not determine the time of onset of puberty. Therefore, impaired GH secretion in children does not cause delayed puberty.

Q: What does deficiency of GH results?
Ans: Neonates: Hypoglycaemia and micropenis
Children: Dwarfism.
Adults: Weight loss, reduced body mass index, lethargy, poor bone density, impaired physical performance in adults, psychological problems, etc.

Q: What makes PRL unique and distinct from the other anterior pituitary hormones?
Ans: Prolactin is a unique hormone because its production is not dependent on a releasing, stimulating, or trophic hormone, as is the case for most of the hormones of anterior pituitary gland.

Q: What are the normal prolactin levels?
Ans: Less than 500 mu/L.

Q: How does secretion of prolactin varies during pregnancy?
Ans: Concentrations rise dramatically during pregnancy. During pregnancy, it is secreted by the decidua in pregnancy. Prolactin is secreted in the middle trimester of pregnancy, and increases progressively towards term.

Q: Is hirsutism a feature of hyperprolactinaemia?
Ans: No, it is not a feature of hyperprolactinaemia because hyperprolactinaemia causes hypogonadism and so does not produce hirsutism per se.

ONE-LINER QUESTIONS

Q: Which dopamine agonist is commonly used for the treatment of hyperprolactinaemia?
Ans: Bromocriptine

Q: What is role of oxytocin?
Ans: 1. Helps in the control of smooth muscle contraction in the uterus.
2. Cause milk release from the lactating breast (the "milk ejection reflex").
3. Primary role of oxytocin is to eject milk from the lactating mammary gland in response to suckling.

Q: What is the use of synthetic oxytocin?
Ans: 1. Induction of labour at term.
2. To produce sustained uterine contractions following delivery (which is required for postpartum or post-termination haemostasis).

Q: What is the plasma half-life of vasopressin?
Ans: Approximately 18 minutes

Q: Which hormone is the primary regulator of body water?
Ans: Vasopressin

Q: What is the location of thyroid gland?
Ans: The thyroid gland is located in the neck at the level of C3 and C4.

Q: Where is T4 converted to T3 and how?
Ans: T4 is converted in some peripheral tissues (liver, kidney, and muscle) to the more active T3 by 5'-monodeiodination.

Q: What is Pendred's syndrome?
Ans: Deficient peroxidase activity associated with a familial goitre and deafness or hearing loss is referred to as Pendred's syndrome.

Q: What are iodine requirements during pregnancy and breastfeeding?

Ans: During pregnancy, 175 µg daily and about 200 µg while breast feeding.

Q: Why does the mother remains euthyroid during pregnancy?
Ans: Although the total amount of T4 is increased in pregnancy, the mother remains euthyroid because the amount of free T4 remains the same.

Q: What is the role of T4 and T3 at the metabolic level?
Ans: They stimulate lipolysis, glycolysis, gluconeogenesis, absorption of glucose, and improved metabolism of cortisol and insulin.

Q: Which is an effective treatment for hyperthyroidism due to Graves' disease or toxic thyroid nodules?
Ans: Radioactive iodine (RAI)

Q: What are the cell types of islets of Langerhans? Which hormones are produced by these cells?
Ans: *Alpha cells*: glucagon
Beta cells: insulin
Delta cells: somatostatin

Q: What conditions result in production of glucagon?
Ans: This hormone is produced in response to hypoglycaemia and the fasting state.

Q: Why is insulin ineffective when taken by the mouth?
Ans: It is ineffective when taken by the mouth because its peptide structure is broken down by digestive proteases in the gut.

Q: How is glycosylated haemoglobin formed?
Ans: It is formed through the non-enzymatic binding of a hexose sugar to the N-terminal amino acid of the β-chain of haemoglobin.

Q: What is the normal level for glycosylated haemoglobin?
Ans: Less than 7%.

Q: What are the precipitating causes of diabetic ketoacidosis?

ONE-LINER QUESTIONS

Ans: Infection, trauma, stroke, pancreatitis, stressful conditions, and inadequate doses of insulin.

Q: What are the lab findings in case of DKA?
Ans: Typical cases of DKA are associated with hyperglycaemia (blood glucose levels greater than 30 mmol/L), presence of ketone bodies in the blood or urine analysis, and acidosis.

Q: What are the lab findings in case of hyperosmolar non-ketotic diabetic coma?
Ans: 1. Absent to low ketonaemia on dipstick
2. Plasma osmolality greater than 320 mOsm/kg
3. Profound dehydration up to an average of 9 L
4. Serum pH greater than 7.3
5. Bicarbonate levels greater than 15 mEq/L
6. Blood sugar level greater than 30 mmol/L

Q: Which cells release testosterone?
Ans: It is released by the Leydig cells of the testes (in response to LH stimulation from the anterior pituitary gland).

Q: Name the three principal androgens in normal women?
Ans: DHT, testosterone, and androstenedione.

Q: What is the function of androgens in female?
Ans: These are responsible for the maintenance of pubic and the axillary hair and also the libido.

Q: Which cells produce follicle-stimulating hormone?
Ans: It is produced by the chromophil cells of the anterior lobe of the pituitary gland.

Q: When does highest pulse frequency and highest pulse amplitude of LH occur?
Ans: The highest pulse frequency of LH occurs during the late luteal phase. Highest pulse amplitude occurs during the early luteal phase.

Q: Which foetal organs are involved in the production of oestriol during pregnancy?
Ans: Large quantities of oestriol are produced during pregnancy. The foetal adrenal and liver are involved in the production of oestriol in conjunction with the placenta.

Q: Which is the major oestrogen formed during pregnancy?
Ans: In pregnancy, the major oestrogen formed is oestriol [due to conversion of the foetal precursor 16-hydroxydehydroepiandrosterone (16OH-DHEA) by the placenta].

Q: Which is the major metabolite of secreted progesterone?
Ans: Pregnanediol glucuronide

Q: How is inhibin produced?
Ans: *Inhibin A*: Dominant follicle, the corpus luteum, and placenta.
Inhibin B: Early follicles

Q: What is the role of prostaglandin F2α and prostaglandin E2 in menstrual cycle?
Ans: Prostaglandin F2α causes myometrial contractions and vasoconstriction. Prostaglandin E2 causes vasodilatation and muscle relaxation.

Q: When does ovulation occurs?
Ans: It takes place on the 14th day of a 28 day cycle, or 14 days before the onset of the next menstrual period. It occurs approximately 34–36 hours after the start of the LH surge or 10–12 hours after the peak of the LH surge.

Q: What is Mittelschmerz syndrome?
Ans: It is the lower abdominal pain, which occurs in the midcycle (experienced by nearly one in four women). This occurs due to ovulation. Rupture of ovum is likely to cause the release of follicular fluid, causing peritoneal irritation.

Q: Which hormone is involved with the "rescue" of the corpus luteum?
Ans: Chorionic gonadotropin (hCG)

ONE-LINER QUESTIONS

Q: What happens to the level of calcium, phosphate and PTH in cases of pseudohypoparathyroidism ?
Ans: Low serum calcium, high serum phosphate, high PTH levels.

Q: What are the characteristics of leptin?
Ans: 1. Acts on the hypothalamus
2. Concentrations are positively correlated with body mass index
3. Concentrations are usually higher in females than males
4. Deficiency is associated with obesity

Q: Which hormone acts on cartilage and liver to release IGF-1?
Ans: Growth hormone

Q: Which is the most characteristic feature of secretory phase of menstrual cycle?
Ans: Development of subnuclear vacuolation in the glandular epithelial cells. In this, the glycogen filled vacuoles are developed between the nuclei and the basement membrane (by the day 17–18). It is the first evidence of occurrence of ovulation.

Q: Which substances are present in reduced concentration in the menstrual fluid?
Ans: Activated prothrombin; antithrombin; antiplasmin; plasminogen; protein C; and factors V, VII, VIII, and X.

Q: What are the four signs of puberty in most adolescent girls?
Ans: 1. An acceleration of growth
2. Breast budding (thelarche)
3. Appearance of pubic hair (pubarche)
4. Onset of menses (menarche).

Q: Which is an important cause of hypogonadotropic hypogonadism?
Ans: Anorexia nervosa.

Q: Who first described physical changes of puberty?
Ans: Marshall and Tanner (known as the Tanner staging system)

Q: What are the changes occurring in vagina at time of puberty?
Ans: 1. A decrease in the vaginal pH
2. Colonisation by Doderlein's bacilli
3. Exfoliation of superficial cells with pyknotic nuclei
4. Glycogenation of the epithelium
5. There are no glands in the epithelium

Q: Define McCune-Albright syndrome.
Ans: Presence of various abnormalities including polyostotic fibrous dysplasia of the skeletal system, patchy cutaneous pigmentation (in form of café-au-lait spots), and precocious pubertal development.

Q: Which is the main cause of delayed puberty?
Ans: The main cause of delayed puberty is hypogonadism. It could be either hypogonadotropic hypogonadism (inactive hypothalamic-pituitary axis) or hypergonadotropic hypogonadism (primary gonadal failure).

Q: Which patients with delayed puberty require diagnostic evaluation?
Ans: The evaluation of delayed puberty is recommended as 13 years in girls and 14 years or older in boys who do not demonstrate any signs of sexual maturation. The first sign of sexual maturity to be considered is thelarche in girls and testicular enlargement in boys.

Q: Which substances are produced by the endometrium during the normal menstrual cycle?
Ans: 1. Endothelins
2. Higher levels of prostaglandins in the secretory phase than in the proliferative phase
3. Increased fibrinolytic activators in the late secretory phase
4. Platelet activating factor (PAF)

Q: Which plasma hormones peak at the middle of a normal menstrual cycle?
Ans. Follicle stimulation hormone

ONE-LINER QUESTIONS

Q: In which conditions raised levels of follicle stimulating hormone are found?
Ans: Gonadal dysgenesis; postmenopausal females; and Turner's syndrome.

Q: Increased motility of the fallopian tube is caused by which hormones?
Ans: Oestrogens

Q: Which cell types are present in the human corpus luteum?
Ans: Endothelial cells; fibroblasts; pericytes; and macrophages.

Q: Which hormone stimulates androgen production from theca cells?
Ans: Luteinising hormone (LH)

Q: Which factors predispose to osteoporosis?
Ans: A sedentary lifestyle; corticosteroid treatment; and heparin therapy.

Q: Features of luteinizing hormone (LH):
Ans: 1. Has a half-life in the circulation of approximately 12 hours
2. Stimulates testosterone production in the male
3. Is released in pulses
4. Plasma concentrations are increased in postmenopausal women

Q: What are the circulating oestradiol level after menopause?
Ans: Approximately 10–20 pg/mL (40–70 pmol/L).

Q: Which was the first SERM used for the treatment of menopausal symptoms?
Ans: Raloxifene

Q: Which hormones are produced by kidneys?
Ans: Erythropoietin; thrombopoietin; renin; 1,25 dihydroxycholecalciferol (calcitriol); and prostaglandins.

Q: What are the causes of hypercalcemia?

Ans: Hyperparathyroidism; vitaminosis D; sarcoidosis; Addison's disease; the milk alkali syndrome; and thyrotoxicosis.

Q: What are the serum calcium levels; serum phosphate; alkaline phosphatase; and parathyroid hormone levels in case of osteoporosis?
Ans: Serum calcium levels: Normal
Serum phosphate: Normal
Alkaline phosphatase: Normal
Parathyroid hormone: Normal

Q: Which pathological conditions lead to secondary hyperparathyroidism?
Ans: Chronic renal failure; vitamin D deficiency; rickets; and impairment of 1-α-hydroxylation of vitamin D by the kidneys.

Q: What are the features of tetany?
Ans: 1. It occurs when serum calcium levels fall below 6 mg/dL.
2. Can be treated with IV calcium gluconate.
3. Skeletal muscle spasms is a main feature of tetany.
4. Treatment can be in the form short-term by slow intravenous injection of calcium ions, e.g. calcium gluconate.
5. This may be treated in the long term by regular doses of vitamin D.

Q: What is the embryological origin of adrenal gland?
Ans: Cortical portion derived from the coelomic epithelium. Medullary portion originally composed of sympathochromaffin tissue.

Q: Which factors regulate aldosterone secretion?
Ans: 1. Increase in potassium ion (K$^+$) concentration in ECF
2. Decrease in sodium ion (Na$^+$) concentration in ECF
3. Decrease in ECF volume (reduced circulating plasma volume, blood loss, hypovolaemia, and hypotension)
4. Increased ACTH secretion

Q: Which biochemical findings are associated with adrenocortical insufficiency?

Ans: Electrolyte imbalance (e.g. hyponatraemia, hyperkalaemia, etc.) and hypoglycaemia acidosis.

Q: Name the common signs and symptoms of Addison's disease.
Ans: Dehydration with loss of sodium, pigmentation of skin and mucous membrane, muscular weakness, hyperkalaemia, decreased cardiac output and decreased workload of the heart, hypotension, hypoglycaemia, dehydration, loss of body weight, nausea, vomiting, diarrhoea, increased susceptibility to any type of infection, inability to withstand any stress, resulting in Addisonian crisis, etc.

Q: What are the characteristic features of Men II syndrome (Wermer's syndrome)?
Ans: Pancreatic tumours such as gastrinomas, insulinomas, VIPomas, glucagonomas, pituitary adenomas, angiofibromas, lipomas, and parathyroid hyperplasia.

Q: How is diagnosis of pheochromocytoma done?
Ans: 1. Presence of elevated levels of free metadrenaline/normetadrenaline in the urine
2. Elevated urinary vanillylmandelic acid (VMA) levels

Q: Which is the most common cause for Addison's disease? What are other causes causing Addison's disease?
Ans: Atrophy of adrenal cortex due to autoimmune diseases. Other causes of Addison's disease include destruction of glands due to tuberculosis, malignancy, etc.

Q: What are the actions of cortisol?
Ans: Anti-inflammation, sodium (and indirectly water) reabsorption, foetal maturation, maintenance of arteriolar tone, insulin antagonism (catabolism), reduced muscle mass, and increased bone resorption.

Last Minute Glances

LAST MINUTE GLANCES
CHAPTER 15
Anatomy

Table 1: Branches of abdominal aorta

Name of the branch	Level of vertebra for origin	Paired or not	Anterior or posterior	Branches
Inferior phrenic artery	T12	Yes	Posterior	

Coeliac axis	Upper L1	No	Anterior	1. Left gastric artery
				2. Splenic artery.
				   ○ Short gastric arteries (six in number)
				   ○ Splenic arteries (six in number)
				   ○ Left gastroepiploic artery
				3. Common hepatic artery
				   ○ Cystic artery
				   ○ Right gastric artery
				   ○ Gastroduodenal artery
				      i. Right gastroepiploic artery
				      ii. Superior pancreaticoduodenal

				artery ○ Right hepatic artery ○ Left hepatic artery

Superior mesenteric artery	Lower Ll	No	Anterior	1. Jejunal and ileal arteries
				2. Inferior pancreaticoduodenal artery
				3. Middle colic artery
				4. Right colic artery
				5. Ileocolic artery
				  a. Anterior caecal artery
				  b. Posterior caecal artery
				  c. Appendicular artery
				  d. Ileal artery
				  e. Colic artery

Middle supra renal artery	L1	Yes	Posterior	
Renal artery	In between L1 and L2	Yes	Posterior	
Gonadal artery	L2	Yes	Anterior	
Lumbar artery	Ll-L4	Yes	Posterior	
Inferior mesenteric artery	L3	No	Anterior	Left colic artery Sigmoid arteries (two or three) Superior rectal artery
Median sacral artery	L4	No	Posterior	
Common iliac artery	L4	Yes	Posterior	External iliac artery Internal iliac artery

Table 2: Different types of pelvis and their characteristics

Characteristic	Gynaecoid (40–50%)	Anthropoid (20%)	Android (30%)	Platypelloid (2–5%)
Pelvic inlet	Oval at the inlet (AP diameter being just slightly less than the transverse diameter)	Oval, long, and narrow. AP diameter of the inlet exceeds the transverse diameter (giving it an oval shape)	Heart shaped/triangular with the base toward the sacrum. Posterior segment is short, and anterior segment is narrow	Pelvic brim: Flat and transverse kidney-shaped. Diameter is much larger than the AP diameter
Bituberous diameter	Normal	Normal or short	Short	Wide
Side wall	Straight	Straight	Convergent side walls	Walls diverge downward
Sacro-sciatic notch	Wide and shallow	Wider and more shallow	Narrow and deep	Slightly narrow and small
Ischial spines	Ischial spines: Not prominent	Ischial spines: Not prominent	Ischial spines: Prominent	Ischial spines: Not prominent
Subpubic arch	Wide and curved subpubic arch Subpubic angle is not <85°	Subpubic arch: Long and narrow Subpubic angle: Slightly narrowed	Subpubic arch: Long and straight Subpubic angle: Narrow	Subpubic arch: Generally wide Subpubic angle is in the excess of 90°

Table 3: Difference between the male and female pelvis

Parameter	Female pelvis	Male pelvis
General structure	Larger and broader	Taller (due to a higher iliac crest), narrower, and more compact
Pelvic canal	Short and almost cylindrical	Long and tape red
Subpubic arch	Wider in females (subpubic angle varying between 90° and 1 00°)	Narrower (subpubic angle varying between 70° and 90°)
Pelvic sidewalls	Wide apart	Sidewall converge from the pelvic inlet towards the outlet
Sacrum	Shorter, wider, and flatter. More curved posteriorly with a less pronounced promontory	Long, narrow, straighter (pronounced sacral promontory)
Pelvic out let	Comparatively large	Comparatively small
Shape of pelvic inlet	Large and oval	Heart shaped
Ischial spines and tuberosity	Less prominent	Heavier (project farther into the pelvic cavity)
Acetabula	Wider and face medially	Narrow and face laterally
Articular surface of the sacrum	Articulates laterally with two sacral bodies; superiorly with L5; oval and occupies one-third of the alar surface	Articulates laterally with three sacral bodies; superiorly with LS and occupies half of the alar surface
Obturator foramen	Triangular	Oval in shape

Table 4: Branches of internal iliac artery

Anterior trunk

Branch	Sub-branch	Area of blood supply
Inferior vesical artery	-	Supplies the prostate, posterior bladder, and seminal vesicle
Superior vesical (umbilical) artery	Umbilical artery may give two vessels: 1. Artery to *vas* deferens 2. Superior vesical artery. (Sometimes, superior vesical artery may branch out directly from the anterior trunk)	Supplies bladder
Middle rectal artery	-	Rectum
Inferior gluteal artery	-	Supply the gluteal muscles
Internal pudendal artery	1. Artery to the bulb of vestibule/bulb of penis 2. Urethral artery 3. Artery of the urethral bulb 4. Inferior rectal artery 5. Perineal artery 6. Posterior labial/scrotal branches 7. Dorsal artery of penis/clitoris 8. Deep artery of the penis/clitoris	Supply the perineum and its muscles, anal canal, bulb of the penis (or vestibule), scrotum (or labia), and urethra
Vaginal artery	-	Vagina
Uterine artery (or the artery of ductus deferens)	Vaginal branch	Uterus

Posterior trunk

Branch	Sub-branch	Area of blood supply
Superior gluteal vessels	-	Supply the gluteal muscles
Iliolumbar vessels	Iliac branches Lumbar branches	Bones and muscles in the iliac Fossa
Lateral sacral vessels	Superior and inferior branches	Branches to the sacrum and coccyx

Table 5: Distinction between the upper and lower areas of the anal canal

Feature for distinction	Above pectinate line	Below pectinate line
Destination of the lymphatic drainage	Internal iliac group of lymph nodes via the pararectal group of lymph nodes	Below the Hilton's line (drainage is to the superficial inguinal group of lymph nodes)
Embryological origin	Endoderm	Ectoderm
Epithelium	Columnar epithelium	Stratified squamous epithelium (non-keratinised until Hilton's line where the anal verge becomes continuous with the perianal skin containing keratinised epithelium)
Nerves	Inferior hypogastric plexus Sympathetic fibres Ll, L2 and parasympathetic fibres S2, S3, S4	Inferior rectal nerves
Artery	Superior rectal artery	Middle and inferior rectal artery
Vein	Superior rectal vein	Middle and inferior rectal vein
Haemorrhoid classification	Internal haemorrhoids (not painful)	External haemorrhoids (painful)

Table 6: Epithelium and its sub-types

System	Tissue	Epithelium	Sub-type
Circulatory	Blood vessels	Simple squamous	Endothelium
Endocrine	Thyroid follicles	Simple cuboidal	-------------
Nervous	Ependyma	Simple cuboidal	------------
Lymphatic	Lymph vessels	Simple squamous	Endothelium
Integumentary	Skin--Dead superficial layers	Stratified squamous, keratinized	-------------
Integumentary	Sweat gland ducts	Stratified cuboidal	-------------
Integumentary	Mesothelium of body cavities	Simple squamous	Mesothelium
Sensory	Cornea	Stratified squamous, non-keratinized	Corneal epithelium
Sensory	Nose	Pseudostratified columnar	Olfactory epithelium

Table 7: Epithelium lining the digestive tract and its sub-types

Tissue	Epithelium	Sub-type
Ducts of submandibular glands	Stratified columnar	-----
Attached gingiva	Stratified squamous, keratinized	-----
Dorsum of tongue	Stratified squamous, keratinized	------
Hard palate	Stratified squamous, keratinized	-------
Oesophagus	Stratified squamous, non-keratinized	--------
Stomach	Simple columnar non-ciliated	Gastric epithelium
Small intestine	Simple columnar non-ciliated	Intestinal epithelium
Large intestine	Simple columnar non-ciliated	Intestinal epithelium
Rectum	Simple columnar non-ciliated	--------
Anus	Stratified squamous, non-keratinized superior to Hilton's white line; Stratified squamous, keratinized inferior to Hilton's white line	--------
Gall bladder	Simple columnar non-ciliated	---------

Table 8: Epithelium lining the urinary tract and its sub-types

Tissue	Epithelium	Sub-type
Kidney—proximal convoluted tubule	Simple cuboidal with microvilli	-------
Kidney—ascending thin limb	Simple squamous	-------
Kidney—distal convoluted tubule	Simple cuboidal with microvilli	-------
Kidney—collecting duct	Simple cuboidal	-------
Renal pelvis	Transitional	Urothelium
Ureter	Transitional	Urothelium
Urinary bladder	Transitional	Urothelium
Prostatic urethra	Transitional	Urothelium
Membranous urethra	Pseudostratified columnar, non-ciliated	-------
Female urethra	Pseudostratified columnar, non-ciliated	-------
External urethral orifice	Stratified squamous	-------

Table 9: Epithelium lining the female reproductive tract and its sub-types

Tissue	Epithelium	Sub-type
Ovaries	Simple cuboidal	Germinal epithelium (Female)
Fallopian tubes	Simple columnar ciliated	-------
Endometrium (uterus)	Simple columnar ciliated	-------
Cervix (endocervix)	Simple columnar	-------
Cervix (ectocervix)	Stratified squamous, non-keratinized	-------
Vagina	Stratified squamous, non-keratinized	-------
Labia majora	Stratified squamous, keratinized	-------

Table 10: Epithelium lining the male reproductive tract and its sub-types

Tissue	Epithelium	Sub-type
Tubuli recti	Simple cuboidal	Germinal epithelium (Male)
Rete testis	Simple cuboidal	-------
Ductus efferentus	Pseudostratified columnar	-------
Epididymus	Pseudostratified columnar with stereocilia	-------
Vas deferens	Pseudostratified columnar	-------
Ejaculatory duct	Simple columnar	-------
Bulbourethral glands	Simple columnar	-------
Seminal vesicles	Pseudostratified columnar	-------

Table 11: Epithelium lining the respiratory tract and its sub-types

Tissue	Epithelium	Sub-type
Oropharynx	Stratified squamous, non-keratinized	-------
Larynx	Pseudostratified columnar, ciliated	Respiratory epithelium
Larynx—True vocal cords	Stratified squamous, non-keratinized	-------
Trachea	Pseudostratified columnar, ciliated	Respiratory epithelium
Respiratory bronchioles	Simple cuboidal	-------

LAST MINUTE GLANCES
CHAPTER 16
Physiology

Table 1: Appearance of centrifuged blood: Clinical significance

Appearance of centrifuged blood	Clinical disorder
Red appearance	Haemolysis
Cloudy milky appearance	High plasma lipid levels
Greatly thickened buffy coat	Leukaemia
Yelllow appearance	Jaundice
Reduced percentage of red blood cells	Anaemia

Table 2: Difference between RBCs and WBCs

Characteristics	RBCs	WBCs
Colour	Red	Colourless
Lifespan	Longer (120 days)	Shorter (12 hours to 15 days
Granules	Absent	Present in some types
Nucleus	Absent	Present
Types	Only one type	Many types (e.g., neutrophils, basophils, eosinophils, monocytes, lymphocytes, etc.)
Shape	Disc-shaped; biconcave	Irregular

Table 3: Life span of different types of WBCs

Type of WBC	Lifespan (days)
Neutrophils	2–5
Lymphocytes	½–1
Eosinophils	7–12
Monocytes	2–5
Basophils	12–15

Table 4: Different types of haemoglobin

Characteristic	Haemoglobin A	Haemoglobin A2	Haemoglobin F
Clinical significance	Main type of haemoglobin in adults	Minor role in normal adults. May assume importance in individuals with chain abnormalities	Main type of haemoglobin in foetus (allowing exchange of gases between placenta and foetal circulation.)
Types of globin chains	Two α chains; two β chains	Two α chains; two δ chains	Two α chains; two γ chains
Proportion of total haemoglobin in a foetus	5–10%	0	90–95%
Proportion of total haemoglobin in an adult	98%	1%	1%
Binding to 2,3-diphosphoglycerate	Binds 2,3-diphosphoglycerate to reduce oxygen affinity	Unable to bind with 2,3-diphosphoglycerate	Unable to bind with 2,3-diphosphoglycerate, so has a higher affinity for oxygen

Table 5: Different waves on ECG trace

ECG Wave	Phase of Cardiac Cycle	Time Duration	Significance
P wave	Atrial depolarization		
PR interval	Depolarization across atrioventricular node Atrial repolarisation occurs during this time.	Normal PR interval 0.12–0.2 seconds	The PR interval is measured from start of the P wave to the start of the QRS complex and serves as a rough approximation of atrioventricular conduction time.
QRS complex	Depolarization of ventricular myocardium	<0.12 seconds	
T wave	Repolarization of ventricular myocardium		Changes in the shape of T wave may occur in different phases of myocardial infraction.
QT interval	It approximates to the ventricular refractory period	0.42 seconds	The QT interval is measured from start of the QRS complex to the end of the T wave.
ST segment	Time period between ventricular depolarisation and ventricular repolarisation		The ST segment is measured from end of the QRS complex to the start of the T wave.

Table 6: Various secretory substances produced by the gastric glands

Cell	*Secretory products*
G-cells	Gastrin
D-cells (delta cells)	Somatostatin
Mucus neck cells	Mucin
Chief cells	Pepsinogen, rennin, gelatinase, lipase, urease
Enterochromaffin cells	Serotonin
Enterochromaffin-like cells	Histamine
Pariietal cellls	Hydrochloric acid Intrinsic factor of Castle

Table 7: Characteristics of different types of jaundice

Features	Pre-hepatic (haemolytic jaundice)	Hepatic (hepatocellular jaundice)	Post-hepatic (Obstructive jaundice)
Cause	Excess breakdown of RBCs	Liver damage	Obstruction of bile ducts
Urinary excretion of urobilinogen	Increases	Decreases	Decreases or is absent in cases of severe obstruction
Faecal excretion of stercobilinogen	Increases	Decreases (pale faeces)	Absent (clay-coloured faeces)
Liver functions	Normal	Abnormal	Exaggerated abnormality
Van den Bergh reaction	Indirect-positive	Biphasic	Direct-positive
Haemorrhagic tendency	Absent	Present (due to lack of vitamin K)	Present (due to lack of vitamin K)
Blood picture	Anaemia, reticulocytosis, abnormal RBCs	Normal	Normal
Plasma albumin and globulin	Normal	Albumin: Decreases Globulin: Normal or increases Albumin:globulin ratio: Decreases	Normal

LAST MINUTE GLANCES

CHAPTER 17
Biochemistry

Table 1: Cytoplasmic organelles with or without a limiting membrane

Organelles with limiting membrane	Organelles without limiting membrane
1. Lysosome 2. Endoplasmic reticulum 3. Centrosome and centrioles 4. Golgi apparatus 5. Nucleus 6. Peroxisome 7. Secretory vesicles 8. Mitochondria	1. Ribosomes 2. Cytoskeleton

Table 2: various types of amino acids in the body

Essential amino acids	Nonessential amino acids
o Valine o Tryptophan o Lysine o Leucine o Isoleuciine o Phenylalanine o Threonine o Methionine o Histidine	o Alanine o Aspartic acid o Asparagine o Arginine o Glutamine o Cysteine o Glutamic acid o Glycine o Proline o Serine o Tyrosine

Table 3: Types of amino acids based on the product of degradation

Glucogenic amino acids	Ketogenic amino acids	Amino acids which are both ketogenic and glucogenic
o Arginine o Asparagine o Aspartate o Glutamate o Glutamine o Histidine o Methionine o Proline o Valine	o Leucine o Lysine o Tryptophan	o Alanine o Cysteine o Glycine o Isoleucine o Phenylalanine o Serine o Threonine o Tyrosine

Table 4: Deficiency disorders

Nutrient substance	Deficiency disorder
Vitamin A	Night blindness, xerophthalmia
Thiamine,	Beriberi
Cyanocobalamin (B12)	Pernicious anaemia, macrocytic anaemia
Niacin (B3)	Pelllagra
Ascorbic acid	Scurvy
Vitamin D	Rickets, osteomalacia

Table 5: Functions of cytoplasmic organelles

Organelles	Functions
Nucleus	o Control of cell division o Control of all the cellular activities o Storage of hereditary information in form of genes present in the DNA o Sending genetic instruction to cytoplasm (for protein synthesis and formation of ribosomal subunits) o RNA synthesis
Golgi apparatus	Processing, packaging, labelling, and delivery of proteins and lipids
RER	o Degradation of worn-out organelles o Synthesis of proteins
SER	o Storage and metabolism of calcium o Synthesis of lipids and steroids o Role in cellular metabolism o Catabolism and detoxification of toxic substances
Centrosome	Movement of chromosomes during cell division
Peroxisomes	o Role in the formation of myelin o Detoxification of hydrogen peroxide and other metabolic products o Oxygen utilisation o Acceleration of gluconeogenesis o Degradation of purine to uric acid o Breakdown of excess fatty acids o Oxygen utilisation o Role in the formation of bile acids
Lysosomes	o Secretion of perforin, granzymes, melanin, and serotonin o Degradation of worn-out organelles o Removal of excessive of secretory products o Degradation of macromolecules
Ribosomes	o Synthesis of proteins
Mitochondria	o Initiation of apoptosis o Synthesis of ATP molecules o Production of energy
Cytoskeleton	o Cellular movements

	<ul><li>Stability of cell shape</li><li>Determination of the cell shape</li></ul>

Table 6: Types of glycogen storage diseases

Type (name of disease)	Type of glycogen storage disease (GSD)	Enzyme which is deficient
Von Geirke's disease	GSD I (type la and lb)	Glucose-6-phosphatase (type la is due to deficiency of the enzyme glucose-6-phosphatase, while type lb is due to the deficiency of a specific translocase Tl which is related with the transport defect of glucose-6-phosphate into the microsomal compartment)
Pompe's disease	GSD II	α-(1,4) glucosidase
Forbe's or Cori's disease or limit dextrinosis	GSD III	Amylo-1, 6-glucosidase, i.e. debranching enzyme
Andersen's disease (amylopectinosis)	GSD IV	1,4 →1,6 *transglucosidase*
McArdle's disease	GSD V	Muscle glycogen phosphorylase
Her's disease	GSD VI	Hepatic phosphorylase
Tauri's disease	GSD VII	Phosphofructokinase

LAST MINUTE RESOURCES FOR MRCOG 1

LAST MINUTE GLANCES
CHAPTER 18
Pathology

Table 1: Difference between acute and chronic inflammation

Feature	Acute inflammation	Chronic inflammation
Definition	Lasts for short duration Within short time	Lasts longer After delay
Plasma exudation	Present	May or may not be present
Cardinal signs	Invariably present	Generally indiscernible
Pathogenesis	Acute inflammatory process is initiated as a result of vascular and cellular events: *Vascular events*: Haemodynamic changes, increased vascular permeability *Cellular events*: Exudation of leucocytes, phagocytosis (mediated via chemical mediators and regulators)	Chronic inflammatory process can occur as a result of the following: Following acute inflammation Recurrent attacks of acute inflammation Chronic inflammation from beginning
Systemic effects	Fever: High grade Leucocytosis (neutrophilic, eosinophilic) Lymphadenitis-lymphangitis Septic shock (in severe acute	Anaemia Amyloidosis (in long-term cases) ESR raised Fever: Mild Leucocytosis (lymphocytic, monocytic)

	infection)	Lymphadenitis-lymphangitis
Main inflammatory cells involved	Neutrophils Lymphomononuclear cells (late) Eosinophils Pus cells	Lymphocytes Monocytes/macrophages (epithelioid cells in granulomas) Plasma cells Giant cells (foreign body, Langhans')
Fate	Chronicity Healing (regeneration, fibrosis) Resolution	Dystrophic calcification Resolution Healing (regeneration, fibrosis)
Main morphology	Ulcers Abscesses (suppuration) Through blood (bacteraemia, septicaemia, and pyaemia)	Granulomatous inflammation (tuberculosis, leprosy, sarcoidosis, syphilis, actinomycosis, Crohn's disease, etc.) Chronic nonspecific inflammation (infectious, others)
Common examples	Cellulitis, pyogenic abscess, bacterial pneumonia, and pyaemia	Granulomatous inflammation (tuberculosis, leprosy, etc.), granulation tissue, and chronic osteomyelitis

Table 2: Difference between metaplasia and dysplasia

Characteristics	Metaplasia	Dysplasia
Definition	One type of differentiated epithelial or mesenchymal cells changes to another type of adult epithelial or mesenchymal cells. Characterised by mature cellular development	It is characterised by disordered cellular development (pleomorphism, nuclear hyperchromasia, mitosis, loss of polarity, etc.). May be accompanied with hyperplasia or metaplasia.
Types	Epithelial (squamous, columnar) Mesenchymal (osseous, cartilaginous)	Epithelial only
Tissues affected	Most commonly affects bronchial mucosa, uterine endocervix; other mesenchymal tissues (cartilage, arteries, etc.)	Uterine cervix, bronchial mucosa
Natural history	Reversible on withdrawal of stimulus	May progress to higher grades of dysplasia or carcinoma in situ. May regress on removal of inciting stimulus

Table 3: Differences between benign and malignant tumours

Characteristics	Benign	Malignant
Size	Usually small	Often larger
Surrounding tissue	Often compressed	Usually invaded
Boundaries	Encapsulated or well-circumscribed	Poorly-circumscribed and irregular
Secondary changes	Occur less commonly	Occur more commonly
Growth rate	Usually slow	Usually rapid
Prognosis	Good (there may be local complications)	Poor (death by local and metastatic complications)
Metastasis	Absent	Frequently present
Local invasion	Often compresses the surrounding tissues without invading or infiltrating them	Usually infiltrates and invades the adjacent tissues
Histopathological pattern	Usually resembles the tissue of origin closely	Often poor resemblance to tissue of origin
Basal polarity	Retained	Often lost
Features of cytological atypia (e.g. pleomorphism, anisonucleosis, hyperchromatism, chromosomal abnormalities, etc.)	Usually absent	Usually present
Nucleocytoplasmic ratio	Normal	Increased
Function	Usually well maintained	May be retained, lost or becomes abnormal
Mitoses	May be present but are always typical mitoses	Mitotic figures increased and are generally a typical and abnormal

Table 4: Causative virus for various cancers

Types of cancer	Causative virus
Hepatocellular carcinoma	o Hepatitis B and C o Exposure to aflatoxin B1 o Alcoholism and haemochromatosis
Kaposi's carcinoma	Human herpes virus 8
Burkitt's lymphoma, Hodgkin's lymphoma, and nasopharyngeal carcinoma	Epstein-Barr virus (human herpes virus 4)
Cervical cancer	o Human papillomavirus subtypes 16 and 18

Table 5: Carcinogen as the likely causative factor for various cancers

Cancer	Carcinogen
Mesothelioma	o Asbestos
Vaginal cell clear cancer	o Exposure to diethylstilbestrol during foetal development
Leukaemia (acute myeloid leukaemia, chronic lymphocytic leukaemia)	o Benzene
Bladder cancer	o Aniline dye (benzidine) o β- naphthylamine (constituent of cigarette smoke)
Bowel cancer	o Low fibre diet, high levels of processed meats, smoking, etc.

Table 6: Underlying pre malignant condition as the likely causative factor for various cancers

Cancer	Underlying pre malignant condition
Oesophageal cancer	Barrett's oesophagus
Cervical cancer	Cervical intraepithelial neoplasia
Squamous cell carcinoma	Actinic keratosis
Gastric adenocarcinoma	Atrophic gastritis
Colorectal cancer	Ulcerative colitis
Oral cancer	Leucoplakia

Table 7: Paraneoplastic syndromes and their associated malignancies

	Paraneoplastic syndrome	*Associated malignancies*	*Mechanism*
Endocrine	Polycythaemia	Kidney, liver and cerebellar haemangioma	Erythropoietin
	Cushing's syndrome	Small cell lung cancer, pancreas, and neural tumours	Production of ACTH or ACTH-like substance
	Hypercalcaemia	Lung (squamous cell carcinoma), kidney, breast and adult T-cell leukaemia, lymphoma	Production of parathormone-like protein, vitamin D
	Hypoglycaemia	Pancreas (islet cell tumour), mesothelioma, and fibrosarcoma	Insulin or insulin-like substance
	Carcinoid syndrome	Bronchial carcinoid tumour, carcinoma pancreas, and stomach	Serotonin, bradykinin
	Syndrome of inappropriate ADH secretion	Lung cancer and tumours of central nervous system	Inappropriate ADH production
Dermatological	Seborrhoeic dermatitis	Bowel	Immunologic
	Dermatomyositis	Breast cancer	Immunologic
	Acanthosis nigricans	Uterine cancer	Immunologic
	Exfoliative dermatitis	Lymphoma	Immunologic

Neuromuscular Syndromes	Neuromuscular disorders	Lung (small cell carcinoma) and breast	Immunologic
	Myasthenia gravis	Thymoma	Immunologic
Osseous, joint, and soft tissues	Hypertrophic osteoarthropathy	Lung	Not known
	Clubbing of fingers	Lung	Not known
Gastrointestinal syndromes	Malabsorption	Lymphoma of small bowel	Hypoalbuminaemia
Renal syndromes	Nephrotic syndrome	Advanced cancers	Renal vein thrombosis, systemic amyloidosis
Hematological	Polycythaemia	Renal cancer and hepatocellular cancer	Increased red cell production
Hematological	Thrombophlebitis (Trousseau's phenomenon)	Pancreas, lung and GIT	Hypercoagulability
	Nonbacterial thrombotic endocarditis	Advanced cancers	Hypercoagulability
	Disseminated intravascular coagulation (DIC)	Acute myeloid leukaemia and adenocarcinoma	Chronic thrombotic phenomena
	Anaemia	Thymoma	Unknown

Table 8: Pathology of various skin lesions

Skin lesion	Description	Disease
Erythema multiforme	Characterised by cutaneous "target" lesions and mucosal involvement	Orf, mycoplasma, and herpes simplex
Erythema nodosum	Tender red swellings usually over the shins	Tuberculosis, sarcoidosis, leprosy, reaction to sulphonamides and inflammatory bowel disease
Erythema marginatum	Non-itchy, pale red, macular eruptions	Major criterion for the diagnosis of rheumatic fever but is also seen in acute glomerulonephritis and drug reactions
Erythema chronicum migrans	An expanding annular lesion	Lyme's disease
Erythema induratum	Nodular eruption usually over the lower legs	Cutaneous tuberculosis (also known as Bazin's disease)

LAST MINUTE GLANCES
CHAPTER 19
Microbiology

Table 1: Common forms of bacteria

Group	Group name	Species	Gram stain	Disease caused
Cocci	Streptococcus (α-haemolytic)	Streptococcus pneumoniae	Positive	Lobar pneumonia
		S. milleri	Positive	Normal flora of the mouth, endocarditis, and deep-seated abscesses
		S. foecalis/Enterococcus foecalis (enterococcus)	Positive	Normal flora of the bowel, urinary tract infection, opportunisitc wound infection, bacteraemia, endocarditis, and abdominal infections
		S. viridans	Positive	Endocarditis, dental caries
	Streptococcus (β-haemolytic)	S. pyogenes(Group A)	Positive	Pharyngitis, upper respiratory tract infection, cellulitis, necrotizing fascitis, pyoderma, erysipelas, rheumatic fever, streptococcal toxic shock syndrome, wound infection, abscesses, bacteraemia, glomerulonephritis, septicaemia, scarlet

				fever, puerperal sepsis, necrotizing fascitis, and septic arthritis
		S. agalactiae (Group B streptococci)	Positive	Normal flora of the vagina, meningitis and chorioamnionitis, neonatal bacteraemia/septicaemia, neonatal sepsis, puerperal fever, meningitis, and pyogenic infection
	Peptostreptococcus	P. anaerobius	Positive	Anaerobic abscesses
	Staphylococcus	S. aureus	Positive	Bacteraemia/septicaemia, Wound infections, abscess, osteomyelitis, TSS, and food poisoning
		S. epidermis	Positive	Vascular cannula-associated infection
		S. saprophyticus	Positive	Urinary tract infections
Cocci	Neisseria	N. gonorrhoeae	Negative	PID, gonorroea, arthritis, neonatal ocular infection, bacteraemia, septicaemia, infertility, and suppurative urethritis (in males)
		N. meningitidis	Negative	Pneumonia, meningitis, bacteriaemia, meningoencephalitis and urethritis

	Moraxellae	*Moraxellae catarrhalis* (Branhamella)	Negative	Respiratory flora, exacerbations of chronic bronchitis
	Veillonella	Veilonella spp.	Negative	Normal oropharyngeal flora
Rods	Nocardia	N. asteroids	Positive	Chronic infection in transplant patients
	Listeria	L. monocytogenes	Positive	Maternal and neonatal listerosis
	Lactobacillus	L. acidophilus	Positive	Normally occurs in the human and animal gastrointestinal tract and mouth
		L. casei	Positive	Normal vaginal flora
	Corynebacterium	C. diphtheriae		Diphtheria
		C. jeikeium		Skin flora. cannula/vascular associated bacteraemia/sepricaemia
	Bacillus	B. anthracis	Positive	Anthrax
		B. cereus	Positive	Food poisoning with diarrhoea and vomiting
	Clostridium	C. perifringens	Positive	Gas gangrene
		C. tetani	Positive	Tetanus
		C. difficile	Positive	Pseudomembranous colitis
	Actinomyces	Actinomyces israelli	Positive	Pelvic actinomycosis
	Mycobacteria	M. tuberculosis	Positive	Tuberculosis

Rods	Enterobacteriaceae			
	Proteus	P. mirabilis		Urinary tract infections
	Escherichia	E. coli	Negative	Urinary tract infections, gastroenteritis
	Klebsiella			
	Salmonella			
	Shigella			
		K. pneumoniae		Pneumonia (bronchopneumonia and bronchitis)
		S. typhi		Enteric fever
		S. dysenteriae		Dysentry
	Pseudomonas	P. aeruginosa	Negative	Nosocomial urinary tract and respiratory tract infection, opportunistic wound infection, bacteraemia, and septicaemia
	Brucella	B. abortus	Negative	Brucellosis or undulant fever
	Bacteroides	B. fragilis	Negative	Intra-abdominal infections perirectal abscess, decubitus ulcer
	Gardernella	G. vaginalis	Negative	Bacterial vaginosis
	Yersinia	Y. pestis	Negative	Plague
		Y. enretocolitica	Negative	Mesenteric adenitis
	Pasteurella	P. multocida	Negative	Animal bites
	Legionella	L. pneumophila	Negative	Atypical pneumonia
	Compylobacter	Compylobacter jejuni	Negative	Gastroenteritis

	Haemophilus	*H. influenzae*	Negative	Respiratory flora, exacerbations of chronic bronchitis
	Bordetella	*B. pertusis*	Negative	Pertussis, whooping cough
	Bartonellae	*B. Henselae*	Negative	Cat-scratch disease. bacillary angiomatosis
Spirochetes	Treponema	*T. palliidum*	Negative	Syphilis
	Leptospira	*L interrogans*	Negative	Leptospirosis
Vibrios	Vibrio (comma-shaped)	*V. cholerae*	Negative	Cholera

Table 2: Diseases caused by spirochaetes

Spirochaete	Species	Diseases	Transmission
Treponema	T. pallidum pallidum	Venereal syphilis	Sexual contact
	T. pallidum endemicum	Endemic syphilis (Bejel)	Mouth to mouth through utensils
	T. pallidum carateum	Pinta	Traumatised skin comes in contact with an infected lesion
	T. pallidum pertenue	Yaws	Traumatised skin comes in contact with an infected lesion
	T. pallidum	Syphilis	Sexual contact or congenital
Leptospira	L. interrogans	Leptospirosis	Rats
Borrelia	B. recurrentis	Epidemic relapsing fever	Body louse
	B. vincentii	Vincent's angina (ulcerative gingivostomatitis or oropharyngitis)	Normal commensal of mouth (which can result in an opportunistic infection)
	B. burgdorferi	Lyme disease	Tick bites (Ixodid ticks)

Table 3: Different types of zoonotic disorders

Type of infection	Examples of the transmitted diseases
Bacterial	o Salmonella food poisoning o Anthrax (cattle and g oats) o Leptospirosis (rats) o Bubonic plague o Brucellosis (sheep) o Bovine tuberculosis (cattle) o Toxocara (cats) o Q fever (cattle, sheep) Listeriosis (pets)
Viral	o Cowpox o Rabies o Monkeypox o Yellow fever
Fungal	o Microsporum canis Trichophyton verrucosum
Protozoan	o Trypanosomiasis o Leishmaniasis o Toxoplasmosis (cats) Babesiosis
Helminthic	o Taeniasis o Echinococcosis Trichinellosis

Table 4: Viruses causing intrauterine infections

Virus infection	Birth defect	Foetal death
Varicella	Yes	Yes
Rubella	Yes	Yes
Cytomegalovirus	Yes	Yes
Poliomyelitis	No	Yes
Japanese B encephalitis	Unknown	
Hepatitis C.	No	Unknown
Hepatitis E	No	Yes
HIV1, HIV2	No	Yes
Coxsackie B virus	No	Yes
Parvovirus B19	No	Yes

Table 5: Risk factors for mother-to-child transmission of HIV

Maternal factors	Obstetric factors
o Low maternal CD4 count o Malnutrition, especially vitamin A deficiency o Advanced maternal disease o Maternal obesity o High maternal viral load o Resistant strain of the virus o Smoking and use of illicit drug o Other sexual transmitted diseases, particularly ulcerative	o Use of scalp electrodes o Episiotomy o Prolonged duration of ruptured membranes o Breastfeeding o Perineal tears and lacerations o Prolonged labour o Chorioamnionitis o Preterm delivery: especially <34 weeks o Active genital ulcer diseaseVaginal delivery

LAST MINUTE GLANCES
CHAPTER 20
Immunology

Table 1: Comparison between active and passive immunity

Characteristics	Active immunity	Passive immunity
Mode of production	Induced by infection or by immunogens	Readymade antibody transferred
Efficacy of the immunity provided	Durable effective protection	Transient, less effective
Participation of the host's immune system	Produced actively by host's immune system	Received passively. No active host participation
Effect of a subsequent dose	Subsequent dose is associated with a booster effect	Subsequent dose less effective
Presence of memory	Immunological memory present	No immunological memory
Time duration for immunity production	Immunity effective only after lag period, i.e. time required for generation of antibodies and immunocompetent cells	Provision of immediate immunity
Occurrence of a negative phase	May occur	Do not occur
Role in immunodeficient individuals	Not applicable	Applicable

Table 2: Various types of antibodies and their properties

Antibody	Function	Characteristic
IgG	Fixes complement; opsonising properties	Produced as a result of the secondary immune response; crosses placenta
IgA	Protection of the mucosal surfaces	Secreted in the saliva, breast milk, tears, etc.
IgM	Fixes complement; opsonising properties	Produced as a result of the primary immune response, i.e. it is a default antibody which is made first in the body
IgE	Activation of the mast cells	Involved in allergic response and anaphylaxis
IgD	Role is uncertain	Found in the serum

Table 3: Different types of vaccines

Type of vaccine	Example
Live-attenuated vaccines • Contain live, but attenuated organisms. • Lack the ability to be pathogenic but are likely to initiate an immune response	1. Herpes zoster (shingles) 2. MMR (Measles, mumps, rubella) 3. Yellow fever (17 D vaccine) 4. Intranasal influenza vaccine (Fluenz®) 5. Bacillus Calmette-Guerin (BCG) 6. Oral typhoid (not used in the UK) 7. Chicken pox 8. Oral polio vaccine (Sabin)
Killed (inactivated) vaccines • Safer than the live vaccines. • Adjuvants such as aluminium hydroxide are added to the killed vaccines in order to precipitate an improved immune response.	1. Injectable typhoid vaccine (available in the UK) 2. Influenza 3. Hepatitis A 4. Pertussis 5. Rabies virus 6. Injectable polio vaccine (Salk vaccine) 7. Cholera vaccine
Toxoid vaccines • Contain a toxin or chemical made by the bacteria or virus (which confers immunity)	1. Tetanus vaccine 2. Diphtheria vaccine
Biosynthetic/conjugate vaccines • Contains manmade substances that are very similar to pieces of the virus or bacteria.	1. The Hib (Haemophilus influenzae type B)
Subunit vaccines Use a specific antigen or purified protein in order to elicit appropriate immune response.	1. Typhoid vaccine (Vi-antigen) 2. Hepatitis B vaccine 3. Hepatitis C vaccine (ongoing research)

DNA vaccines Genes for the microbe's antigens are introduced into the body (which is taken up by some cells) DNA instructs those cells to make antigen molecules (thereby invoking the immune response)	1. Vaccine against the West Nile Virus
Recombinant vector vaccines An attenuated virus or bacterium is used to introduce the microbial DNA into the body cells. This causes the formation of antigen molecule and thus stimulates the body's immune mechanism. Vector is the virus or bacteria used as a carrier.	1. There is an ongoing research for recombinant vector vaccines against diseases such as rabies, HIV, and measles

LAST MINUTE GLANCES
CHAPTER 21
Embryology

Table 1: Site of synthesis of various hormones

Hormone	Site of synthesis
Prolactin	Anterior pituitary gland
Testosterone	Testis (Leydig cells)
17-alpha-hydroxyprogesterone	Adrenal gland
Oestradiol	Testis (Leydig cells)
Inhibin	Sertoli cells

Table 2: Fate of germ layers

Germ layer	Structures derived
Endoderm	Epithelial lining of: o Respiratory o Gastrointestinal tract
Mesoderm	o Connective tissues, vessels, and skeleton o Reproductive/excretory organs o Cardiovascular system Smooth and striated muscles
Ectoderm	o Neuroectoderm: CNS, PNS, neural crest cells, and derivatives Surface ectoderm: Epidermis, and other external structures

Table 3: Different types of arches and their derivatives

Name of the arch	Post-trematic nerve	Muscles/bones derived
First pharyngeal arch/mandibular arch	Mandibular branch of trigeminal nerve (5th cranial nerve)	1. Anterior belly of digastric 2. Mylohyoid 3. Tensor tympani, Tensor palati, lateral, and medial pterygoid 4. Muscles of mastication 5. Tensor palati and tympani muscles 6. Masseter, temporalis, stylohyoid, and anterior belly of digastric 7. Skeletal derivatives: incus, malleus, part of the mandible, sphenomandibular ligament, and zygomatic bone
Second pharyngeal arch/hyoid arch	Facial (7th cranial nerve)	1. Muscles of auricle 2. Muscles of facial expression: orbicularis oris and occuli, platysma, buccinator, and frontalis 3. Occipitofrontalis, platysma 4. Stapedius, stylohyoid ligament 5. Posterior belly of

		digastric 6. Skeletal derivative: stapes
Third arch	Glossopharyngeal nerve	Stylopharyngeus
Fourth arch	Superior laryngeal nerve	Muscles of soft palate, pharynx, and cricothyroid
Fifth arch disappears		
Sixth arch	Recurrent laryngeal nerve	Muscles of larynx (except cricothyroid)

CHAPTER 22
Genetics

Table 1: Diseases showing autosomal recessive pattern of inheritance

- Alpha 1-antitrypsin deficiency
- Alpha thalassemia
- Adrenogenital syndrome
- Beta thalassemia
- Cystic fibrosis
- Familial Mediterranean Fever
- Familial hypercholesterolaemia
- Friedreich's Ataxia
- Galactosaemia
- Gaucher's Disease
- Homocystinuria
- Hurler's syndrome
- Sickle cell disease
- Phenylketonuria
- 21-hydroxylase deficiency
- Mucopolysaccharidoses
- Glycogen storage disease
- Tay-Sachs disease
- Galactosaemia
- Wilson's disease
- Hemochromatosis

Table 2: Diseases showing X-linked recessive pattern of inheritance

- Adrenoleukodystrophy
- Becker's Muscular Dystrophy
- Both haemophilias A and B
- Colour blindness
- Duchenne's Muscular dystrophy
- Fragile X syndrome
- Glucose-6-phosphate dehydrogenase (G6PD) deficiency
- Kallmann's syndrome
- Nephrogenic diabetes insipidus (Autosomal recessive in some cases)
- Vitamin D resistant rickets

Table 3: Diseases showing autosomal dominant pattern of inheritance

- Adult polycystic kidney disease (ADPKD)
- Achondroplasia
- Basal cell nevus syndrome
- Dystrophia Myotonica (variable penetrance)
- Familial adenomatous polyposis
- Huntington's Chorea
- Familial hypercholesterolaemia (FH)
- Familial breast and ovarian cancer
- Familial melanoma
- Factor V Leiden
- Neurohypophyseal diabetes insipidus
- Maturity onset diabetes of the Young
- Marfan's syndrome
- Hypokalemic periodic paralysis
- Acute intermittent porphyria
- Primary Pulmonary hypertension
- Retinoblastoma
- Neurofibromatosis
- Polyposis coli
- Multiple endocrine neoplasia (MEN) type 1
- Spinocerebellar ataxia
- Hereditary non-polyposis colon cancer
- Malignant hyperthermia
- Long QT syndrome
- Hypertrophic cardiomyopathy
- Familial hypocalciuric hypercalcaemia
- Polycystic kidney disease
- Familial Parkinson's Disease
- Malignant hyperthermia
- Alzheimer's disease (some cases)

Table 4: Karyotype abnormalities in some common chromosomal disorders

Chromosomal disorder	Karyotype abnormality
Cri du chat syndrome	Deletion on chromosome 5p
Down syndrome	Trisomy 21
Edward's syndrome	Trisomy 18
Klinefelter's syndrome	47,XXY
Patau's syndrome	Trisomy 13
Turner's syndrome (gonadal dysgenesis)	XO
Testicular feminisation syndrome	46,XY

Table 5: Common syndromes caused by chromosomal microdeletions

Chromosomal disorder	Chromosomal microdeletion
Angelman syndrome	Microdeletion associated with the loss of maternally inherited chromosome 15
Cri du chat syndrome	Deletion on the short arm of chromosome 5
Di-George syndrome, Shprintzen syndrome	Deletion of the proximal long arm of chromosome 22
Prader-Willi syndrome	Microdeletion associated with the loss of paternally inherited chromosome 15
Smith-Magenis syndrome	Microdeletion affecting chromosome 17
Williams syndrome	Microdeletion affecting chromosome 7

LAST MINUTE GLANCES

CHAPTER 23

Biophysics

Table 1: Different types of ultrasound signals

Type of ultrasound signal	Definition
A-mode (amplitude)	o Echo is displayed in form of a deflection (spike) on oscilloscope (as the ultrasound wave comes in contact with various tissues) o Size of the wave spike is related to the strength of the echo. o Rarely used nowadays
B-mode (brightness)	o Movement of the transducer yields a series of dots. o This results in a two-dimensional image (brightness modulation)
Gray-scale ultrasound	o Selective amplification of low-level echoes from the soft tissue
Real-time	o Successive B-scans are generated by movement of transducer automatically either mechanically or via electronic means
M-mode (time-position mode)	o Continuous displacement of B scan with respect to the time. o It demonstrates movement
Doppler mode	o Used for assessing movement o Can be used for looking at the blood flow

Table 2: Side effects of radiotherapy

Acute	Late
Cystitis	Further development of cancers
Epithelial surface damage (e.g. mouth ulcerations)	Lymphoedema
Fatigue	Tissue fibrosis
Gastrointestinal damage. Results in symptoms: • Nausea • Vomiting • Abdominal pain	Hair loss
Oedema	Infertility

Table 3: Equivalent duration of natural background radiation of various imaging modalities

Imaging modality	Equivalent duration of natural background radiation
Chest X-ray	2–10 days
CT abdomen	3 years
Intravenous urogram	1 year
X-ray lumbar spine	6 months

LAST MINUTE GLANCES
CHAPTER 24
Epidemiology

Table 1: Simple formulas for calculating the sensitivity, specificity, positive predictive value and the negative predictive value

	Disease present	Disease absent	
Test positive	a (true positive)	b (false positive)	a + b
Test negative	c (false negative)	d (true negative)	c + d
	a + c	b + d	a + b + c + d

a = true positives (Persons who have disease and are test positive on the screening test)
b = false positives (Persons who do not have disease and test positive on the screening test)
c = false negatives (Person with disease but with negative test)
d = true negatives (Persons who do not have disease and are test negative)
Sensitivity = a/ a + c (Ability of the test to be correctly positive amongst those who are known to have the disease)
Specificity = d / b + d (Ability of the test to be correctly negative among those who are known to be without disease)
Positive predictive value= a/ a + b (Ability of the test to correctly predict presence of the disease)
Negative predictive value = d / c + d (Ability of the test to correctly predict the absence of disease)

Table 2: Methodology for data measurement

Continuous data	*Categorical data*
Single group 1. Normally distributed: Mean, standard deviation, 95% confidence interval 2. Non-normal: Median, range, interquartile range	Single group 1. Rate (risk) 2. 95% confidence interval
Two groups 1. Mean difference 2. 95% confidence interval	Two groups 1. Risk difference, 95% confidence interval 2. Relative risk, 95% confidence interval 3. Odds ratio, 95% confidence interval

CHAPTER 25
Pharmacology

Table 1: Drugs inhibiting and inducing hepatic microsomal enzymes

Enzyme inducers	Enzyme inhibitors
o Barbiturates o Carbamazepine o Ethanol (chronic) o Griseofulvin o Phenytoin o Phenobarbitone o Rifampicin	o Amiodarone o Cimetidine o Ciprofloxacin o Erythromycin o Ethanol (acute) o Fluconazole o Ketoconazole o Metronidazole

Table 2: Classification of antipsychotic drugs

- *Atypical antipsychotics:* Aripiprazole, clozapine, risperidone, olanzapine, ziprasidone, etc.
- *Butyrophenones:* Haloperidol, penfluridol, and trifluperidol
- *Phenothiazines:* Chlorpromazine, fluphenazine, triflupromazine, thioridazine, trifluoperazine, etc.
- *Thioxanthenes:* Flupenthixol
- *Other heterocyclics:* Pimozide, loxapine

Table 3: Classification of narcotic (opioid) analgesic drugs

- *Natural opium alkaloids:* Codeine, Morphine
- *Semisynthetic opiates:* Diacetylmorphine (Heroin), ethylmorphine, hydrocodone, hydromorphone, oxymorphone, pholcodine, etc.
- *Synthetic opioids:* Dextropropoxyphene, fentanyl, methadone, pethidine (meperidine), and tramadol.

Table 4: Drugs interfering with glucose metabolism

Drugs causing hyperglycaemia	Drugs causing hypoglycaemia
o Corticosteroids o Glucagon o Thiazide diuretics	o Aspirin o Atenolol o Ethanol o Gliclazide

Table 5: Classification of antiemetic agents

Adjuvant antiemetics
o Benzodiazepines o Chlorpropamide o Cyclizine o Dexamethasone
Anticholinergics
o Hyoscine o Dicyclomine
5-HT3 antagonists
o Ondansetron o Granisetron
H1 antihistaminics
o Cinnarizine o Diphenhydramine o Dimenhydrinate o Doxylamine o Meclozine (Meclizine) o Promethazine
Neuroleptics (D2 blockers)
o Chlorpromazine o Droperidol o Haloperidol o Perphenazine o Prochlorperazine o Triflupromazine

Prokinetic drugs
o Cisapride o Domperidone o Metoclopramide

Table 6: Different types of antihypertensive agents

Drug	Mechanism of Action
Alpha-methyldopa	A centrally acting sympathomimetic agent
Carvedilol	Combined alpha- and beta-blocking effects
Captopril	Angiotensin converting enzyme inhibition
Hydralazine hydrochloride	Directly acting vasodilator
Losartan, eprosartan, and irbesartan	Blockade of the angiotensin II receptor
Propranolol/Atenolol	Non-selective beta-receptor antagonist
Prazosin and doxazosin	Specific alpha-1-recept or antagonist
Phentolamine	Alpha-adrenoceptor blockade
Sodium nitroprusside	Vasodilatation
Verapamil	Calcium antagonist

Table 7: Mechanism of action of various antibiotics

Mode of action	Antibiotic
Causing leakage from cell membranes	o Polypeptides—polymyxins, colistin, and bacitracin o Polyenes—amphotericin b, nystatin, and hamycin
Causing misreading of m-RNA code and effect on permeability	Aminoglycosides—streptomycin, gentamicin, etc.
Inhibition of cell wall synthesis	Penicillins, cephalosporins, cycloserine, vancomycin, bacitracin
Inhibition of protein synthesis	Tetracyclines, chloramphenicol, erythromycin, clindamycin, and linezolid
Inhibition of nucleic acid synthesis	Metronidazole
Inhibition of DNA gyrase	Fluoroquinolones—ciprofloxacin and others
Interference with DNA function	Rifampin
Interference with DNA synthesis	Acyclovir, zidovudine
Interference with intermediary metabolism	Sulphonamides, sulphones, PAS, trimethoprim, pyrimethamine, and metronidazole

Table 8: Classification of antibiotics based on the type of action

Primarily bacteriostatic	Primarily bactericidal
o Chloramphenicol o Clindamycin o Erythromycin o Ethambutol o Linezolid o Sulphonamides o Tetracyclines	o Aminoglycosides o Ciprofloxacin o Cephalosporins o Cotrimoxazole o Isoniazid o Metronidazole o Penicillins o Polypeptides o Pyrazinamide o Rifampin o Vancomycin

Table 9: Different generations of cephalosporins

First generation cephalosporins	
Parenteral	*Oral*
o Cefazolin	o Cefadroxil o Cephalexin
Second generation cephalosporins	
Parenteral	*Oral*
o Cefoxitin o Cefuroxime	o Cefaclor o Cefprozil o Cefuroxime axetil
Third generation cephalosporins	
Parenteral	*Oral*
o Cefoperazone o Cefotaxime o Ceftriaxone o Ceftizoxime o Ceftazidime	o Cefetamet pivoxil o Cefdinir o Cefixime o Cefpodoxime proxetil o Ceftibuten
Fourth generation cephalosporins	
	Parenteral
	o Cefpirome o Cefepime

Table 10: Characteristics of local anaesthetic agents

Name of the local anaesthetic	Properties
Bupivacaine	o Most widely used drug in epidural anaesthesia o Duration of 2–3 hours o Used at strength of 0.25% (although higher concentrations may be used) o Highly protein-bound (thereby associated with limited transplacental exchange) o Action starts slowly (within 30 minutes) but lasts for a longer duration of time (8 hours)
Benzocaine	o Weak agent used for providing surface analgesia in mouth and anus
Mepivacaine	o Does not cause vasodilatation and is therefore used in spinal anaesthesia.
Ropivacaine	o Newer bupivacaine congener (equally long-acting but less cardiotoxic) Continuous epidural ropivacaine is being used for relief of postoperative and labour pain. o Employed for nerve blocks.

Table 11: Drugs likely to have deleterious effects during lactation

- Amantadine
- Amiodarone
- Antineoplastic drugs
- Atropine
- Barbiturates
- Benzodiazepines
- Bromide
- Carbimazole
- Chloramphenicol
- Ephedrine
- Ergotamine
- Iodide
- Lithium
- Phenindione
- Primidone
- Radioactive agents
- Streptomycin
- Sulphonamides

Chapter 26
Obstetrics

Table 1: Investigations that suggests persistent gestational trophoblastic disease

- Choriocarcinoma proved on histopathological studies
- Increase in β-hCG levels over two samples
- β-hCG levels more than 20,000 IU/L even 4 weeks after the uterus was emptied
- Elevation of hCG level and hitting a plateau over three samples
- Evidence suggests of metastases
- Heavy bleeding and elevated hCG levels

Table 2: Features suggestive of poor prognosis choriocarcinoma

- Advanced maternal age
- Large or multiple secondaries (especially in liver, bowel, and brain)
- Type of antecedent pregnancy (choriocarcinoma which follows a normal pregnancy has a worse prognosis than that which follows a mole)
- Failure of preliminary drug therapy
- High levels of hCG (reflects high residual tumour loads)
- Blood groups B and AB
- Interval between the diagnosis and the antecedent pregnancy is long

Table 3: WHO criterion for 75 g oral glucose tolerance test

	Whole blood (venous)	Whole blood (capillary)	Plasma (venous)	Plasma (capillary)
Fasting	≥ 6.11 mmol/L	≥ 6.1 mmol/L	≥ 7.0 mmol/L (126 mg/dL)	≥ 7.0 mmol/L
2 hours	≥ 6.7 mmol/L	≥ 6.7 mmol/L	≥ 7.8 mmol/L (140 mg/dL)	≥ 8.9 mmol/L

Table 4: Blood indices abnormalities with iron deficiency anaemia

Blood index	Normal value	Value in iron deficiency anaemia
Haemoglobin	12.1–14.1 g/dL	<11 g/dL in 1st and 3rd trimesters. and less than 10.5 g/dL in 2nd trimester
Haematocrit	36.1–44.3%	<36.1%
Mean corpuscular haemoglobin concentration	32–36 g%	<30g%
Mean corpuscular volume	83–97 fL (average 90 fL)	<76 fL
mean corpuscular haemoglobin	26.7–33.7 pg/cell (average 30.6 pg/cell)	<26.7 pg/cell
Red cell count	3.9–5.0 × 10^6 cells/L	<3.9 × 10^6 cells/µL (or normal)
Red cell distribution index	31–36%	<31%

Table 5: Classification of anaemia on the basis of blood values

Macrocytic normochromic anaemia	MCHC normal (MCHC-34) MCV increased (MCV >100 fL	Folate deficieny anaemia Vitamin 12 deficiency
Microcytic hypochromic anaemia	MCHC low (MCHC <30) MCV low (MCV <80 fL)	Anaemia of chronic disease (rare cases) Thalassemia Iron deficiency anaemia
Normocytic normochromic anaemia	MCHC normal MCV normal	Anaemia due to chronic disease Anaemia due to acute haemorrhage Aplastic anaemia Physiological anaemia of pregnancy Haemolytic anaemia

Abbreviations: MCV, mean corpuscular volume; MCHC, mean corpuscular haemoglobin concentration

Table 6: Difference between monozygotic and dizygotic twins

Parameter	Monozygotic twins (Identical twins)	Dizygotic twins (non-identical or fraternal twins)
Incidence	Comprises of one-third of total cases of twins	Comprises of two-third of total cases of twins
Aetiology	Division of a fertilised ovum into two	Fertilisation of two or more ova by sperms
Sex	Same	Can be different
Placenta	Single	Each foetus has a separate placenta
Intervening membrane between the two foetuses	Composed of three layers: a fused chorion in the middle surrounded by amnion on two sides	Composed of four layers: two chorions in the middle surrounded by amnion on two sides
Genetic features (DNA fingerprinting)	Same	Different
Skin grafting	Acceptance by the other twin	Rejection by the twin
Blood group	Same	Different
Foetal growth and congenital malformations	More common	Less common
Communication between foetal vessels	Present	Absent

Table 7: Complications related to pre-eclampsia

Maternal	Foetal
o Abruption placenta o Cerebral haemorrhage o Eclampsia o HELLP syndrome o Impaired renal/liver function tests o Maternal death o Pre-eclampsia in subsequent pregnancies o Pulmonary oedema	o Intrauterine asphyxia and acidosis o Intrauterine death Oligohydramnios o IUGR o Premature delivery (before 37 weeks of gestation) o Pre-eclampsia in subsequent pregnancies o Infant death

Table 8: Degree of polyhydramnios

Grading	Criteria
Mild	Measurement of largest vertical pocket of liquor 8–11 cm
Moderate	Measurement of largest vertical pocket of liquor 12–15 cm
Severe	Measurement of largest vertical pocket of liquor >16 cm

Table 9: APGAR score

Feature	Score = 0	Score = 1	Score = 2
Appearance	White	Blue	Pink
Pulse	0	<100	100 or more
Grimace (reflex irritability)	None	Grimace	Cry
Activity (Muscle tone)	Limp	Some flexion of the extremities	Active movement (good flexion)
Respiration	Absent	Gasping/weak cry	Regular/good cry

Table 10: Bishop's score (modified)

Score	Dilation (cm)	Effacement (%)	Station of the presenting part	Cervical consistency	Position of cervix
0	Closed	0–30	–3	Firm	Posterior
1	1–2	40–50	–2	Medium	Mid position
2	3–4	60–70	–1,0	Soft	Anterior
3	>5	>80	+1,+2	–	–

Table 11: Stages of labour

Stages	Description	Characteristics	Duration (in primigravida)	Duration (in multigravida)
Stage I	Starts: From the onset of true labour pains Ends: With the complete dilatation of the cervix	Two phases: *Latent phase:* Cervical effacement is slow and gradual Dilatation (up to 3 cm) *Active phase:* Active cervical dilatation (3–10 cm) and foetal descent. It consists of three phases: <ul><li>Acceleration phase</li><li>Phase of maximum slope</li><li>Deceleration phase</li></ul>	-	-
Stage II	Starts: From full dilatation of cervix Ends: With expulsion of the foetus from birth canal	-	50 min	20 min
Stage III	Starts: After	-	15 min	15 min

	expulsion of the foetus Ends: With expulsion of placenta and membranes			
Stage IV	Stage of observation: Starts: After the expulsion of afterbirths	-		60 min	60 min

LAST MINUTE GLANCES
CHAPTER 27
Gynaecology

Table 1: Causes of primary amenorrhoea

- Androgen insensitivity: XY female or testicular feminisation.
- Genitourinary malformation, e.g. imperforate hymen, transverse vaginal septum, absent vagina with or without a functioning uterus
- Mullerian agenesis (Mayer Rokitansky Küster-Hauser syndrome)
- Gonadal failure, e.g. ovarian dysgenesis/agenesis, premature ovarian failure
- Gonadotropin deficiency, e.g. Kallmann's syndrome
- Hyperprolactinaemia
- Hypothalamic dysfunction, e.g. chronic illness, anorexia, weight loss, stress
- Hypothyroidism
- Tumours of the hypothalamus or pituitary gland
- Hypopituitarism
- Resistant ovary syndrome

Table 2: Causes of secondary amenorrhoea

- Anorexia nervosa
- Asherman's syndrome
- Congenital hypothyroidism
- Following surgical procedures of cervix (e.g. cervical stenosis)
- Hyperprolactinaemia
- Thyrotoxicosis
- Use of LH-RH analogues
- Virilising ovarian tumours

Table 3: Normal parameters for semen analysis (World Health Organization, 4th Edition, 1999)

Parameter	Normal range
Volume	2–5 ml
Sperm morphology	>50% normal (WHO,1987, 2nd Edition) >30% normal (WHO,1992, 3rd Edition) >14% normal (WHO,1999, 4th Edition)
Liquefaction	Complete in 30 minutes
Sperm density	>20 million spermatozoa per ml or more
Total sperm number	40 million spermatozoa per ejaculate or more
Motility	50% (forward progression) 50% or more motile (grades a* and b**) 25% or more with progressive motility (grade a) within 60 minutes of ejaculation
WBC	<1 million/ml
Immunobead test	<20% spermatozoa with adherent particles
Spermmar test	<10% spermatozoa with adherent particles

*Grade a: Rapid progressive motility (sperm moving swiftly, usually in a straight line)

**Grade b: Slow or sluggish progressive motility (sperms may be less linear in their progression)

Table 4: Parameters for semen analysis: lower reference limits (95% CI) in fertile men (World Health Organization, 5th Edition, 2010)

Parameter	Normal range
Volume	1.5 mL (1.4 mL–1.7 mL)
Sperm concentration	15 (12–16) million/mL or greater
Total sperm number	39 (33–46) million spermatozoa per ejaculate or more
Motility	32%, forward progression; 40% total motility (progressive + nonprogressive motility)
Sperm morphology	Normal sperms (> 4%) using "strict" Tygerberg method
Vitality	58 (55–63)% or more live

Table 5: Causes of male infertility

- Environmental factors: Exposure to chemicals (lead, nickel, mercury, anaesthetic agents, pesticides, tobacco smoking, excessive alcohol intake, etc.)
- Idiopathic.
- Genetic and endocrine disorders (Klinefelter's syndrome, androgen insensitivity syndrome, disorders of pituitary and adrenal glands, adrenal hyperplasia)
- Infections
  - Acute systemic infections (smallpox, mumps, other viral infections)
  - Chronic systemic infections (TB, leprosy, filariasis, prostatitis, renal, hepatic diseases, diabetic neuropathy)
  - STDs (Chlamydia, gonorrhoea, syphilis)
- Undescended testes (cryptorchidism)
- Varicocoele
- Excessive intake of alcohol and/or drugs
- Torsion, undescended testes; damage to the testis due to exercise or heat; tumours (seminoma); and hydrocele.
- Long-term use of drugs: Anti-hypertensive drugs (anabolic steroids, antipsychotics, cimetidine, guanethidine, reserpine, methyldopa, pironolactone, propranolol, corticosteroids, and certain anti-cancer drugs)
- Previous surgery: Inguinal, scrotal, retroperitoneal, bladder neck, vasectomy, hernia repair, etc.
- Sexual dysfunctions: Ejaculatory disturbances, impotence, etc.

Table 6: Causes of female fertility

Cervical factor infertility
- Abnormalities of the mucus-sperm inter action
- Narrowing of the cervical canal due to cervical stenosis

Ovarian factor infertility
- Polycystic ovarian syndrome

Uterine factor infertility
- Total absence of the uterus and vagina (Rokitansky-Kuster-Hauser syndrome)
- Diethylstilbestrol-induced uterine malformations
- Asherman's syndrome, endometritis (due to tuberculosis)
- Leiomyomas

Tubal factors
- Pelvic inflammatory disease associated with gonorrhoeal and chlamydial infection

Peritoneal factors
- Infection
- Adhesions and adnexal masses
- Endometriosis

Table 7: Indications of various surgeries performed for uterine prolapse

Anterior Colporrhaphy
- Presence of cystocoele, urethrocoele, or a cystourethrocoele
- Repair of anterior defects

Hysterectomy
- Concomitant uterine or cervical pathology (e.g. large fibroid uterus, endometrial carcinoma, etc.)
- Patient desires removal of the uterus
- Removal of a non-functioning organ in postmenopausal women

Le Fort Colpocleisis
- No sexual activity at present or no plans for sexual activity in future
- Patient is medically fragile.

Manchester Operation
- Absence of UTI
- Absence of an enterocoele
- Childbearing function is not required.
- Malignancy of the endometrium has been ruled out.
- Patient requires preservation of menstrual function.
- Presence of a small cystocoele with only a first- or second-degree prolapse
- Symptoms of prolapse are largely due to cervical elongation.

Posterior Colpoperineorrhaphy
- Presence of a rectocoele
- Repair of posterior defects

Table 8: Diagnostic features of the commonest causes of vaginitis

Basis of diagnosis	Bacterial vaginosis	Vulvovaginal candidiasis	Trichomoniasis
Signs and symptoms	Thin, greyish to off-white coloured discharge Unpleasant "fishy" odour especially increasing after sexual intercourse Discharge is usually homogeneous and adheres to vaginal walls	Thick, white (curd-like) discharge No odour	Copious, malodorous, yellow-green (or discoloured) discharge Pruritus, vaginal irritation, and dysuria Asymptomatic in many cases
Vaginal pH	Elevated (> 4.5)	Normal	Elevated (> 4.5)
"Whiff" test (Normal = no odour)	Positive	Negative	Can be positive
Physical examination	Greyish white-coloured discharge (may be adherent to the vaginal walls) Normal appearance of vaginal	Thick white discharge that adheres to the vaginal walls Vulvar and vaginal erythema, oedema, and fissures	Frothy purulent discharge "Strawberry" cervix in up to 25% of affected women Vulvar and vaginal oedema and erythema

	tissues		
Microscopic examination of wet-mount and KOH preparations of the vaginal discharge	"Clue cells" (vaginal epithelial cells coated with coccobacilli) Few lactobacilli Occasional motile, curved rods (belonging to preparations of Mobiluncus species)	Budding yeast cells Mycelial tangles Pseudo-hyphae	Motile trichomonads Many polymorphonuclear cells

LAST MINUTE GLANCES
CHAPTER 28
Endocrinology

Table 1: Various hormones produced in the body by the endocrine glands

Name of endocrine gland	Hormones produced
Hypothalamus	o Corticotropin-releasing hormone (CRH) o Dopamine (prolactin inhibiting hormone) o Gonadotropin-releasing hormone (GnRH) o Growth hormone-releasing hormone (GHRH) o Somatostatin (growth hormone-inhibiting hormone) o Thyrotropin-releasing hormone (TRH)
Anterior pituitary	o Adrenocorticotropic hormone (ACTH) o Follicle-stimulating hormone (FSH) o Growth hormone (GH) o Luteinising hormone (LH) o Prolactin o Thyroid-stimulating hormone (TSH)
Posterior pituitary	o Antidiuretic hormone (ADH) o Oxytocin
Thyroid gland	o Calcitonin o Thyroxine (T4) o Triiodothyronine (T3)
Parathyroid gland	o Parathormone

Pancreas (Islets of Langerhans)	o Insulin o Glucagon o Pancreatic polypeptide o Somatostatin
Adrenal cortex	o Mineralocorticoids o Aldosterone o 11-deoxycorticosterone o Glucocorticoids o Cortisol o Corticosterone o Sex hormones o Androgens o Oestrogen o Progesterone
Adrenal medulla	o Adrenaline (Epinephrine) o Catecholamines o Dopamine o Noradrenaline (Norepinephrine)

Table 2: Characteristic features of diabetic ketoacidosis

o Increased carbon dioxide partial pressure (pCO_2) o Increased plasma glucose levels o Leucocytosis o Reduced levels of bicarbonate o Reduced pH o Reduced oxygen partial pressure (pO_2)

Table 3: Substances present in reduced concentration in the menstrual fluid

o Activated prothrombin o Antithrombin o Antiplasmin o Factors V, VII, VIII, and X o Plasminogen o Protein C

Table 4: Tanner stages of breast development

Stage	Characteristic features
Stage 1	Prepubertal stage age 10 and younger
Stage 2	Breast bud forms Enlargement and widening of the areolae Age 10–11.5
Stage 3	Breast enlargement beyond the areolae Age 11.5–13
Stage 4	Further enlargement of the breasts Areolae and nipples form the secondary mounds Age 13–15
Stage 5	Adult breast contour Age 15+

Table 5: Tanner stages of pubic hair development

Stage	Characteristic features
Stage 1	Prepubertal hair: no hair Age 10 and younger
Stage 2	Presexual hair Long, relatively straight hair on labia majora Age 10–11.5
Stage 3	Sexual hair Hair becomes curly, coarser and there is an lateral extension Age 11.5–13
Stage 4	Mid-escutcheon Extension of the hair to cover the labia Age 13–15
Stage 5	Female escutcheon Extension of hair over the medial thighs Age 15+

Table 6: Symptoms of phaeochromocytoma

- Anxiety
- Chest pain
- Diarrhoea
- Fever, sweats
- Headache
- Hypertension (also known as endocrine or secondary hypertension)
- Hyperglycaemia
- Metabolic disorders
- Nausea and vomiting
- Palpitation
- Paroxysmal panic attacks
- Polyuria and glucosuria
- Sweating and flushing
- Tachycardia
- Tremor
- Weight loss

Table 7: Immediate, intermediate, and long-term effects of menopause

Immediate effects	Intermediate effects	Long-term effects
1. Cognitive dysfunction: Poor concentration, memory loss, loss of motivation, tiredness, etc. 2. Insomnia 3. Mood swings: Irritability, depression, anxiety 4. Sexual dysfunction: Dyspareunia and reduced libido 5. Reduction of the rapid eye movement (REM) sleep time 6. Urinary symptoms: Recurrent urinary tract infection, dysuria, lower urgency, etc. 7. Vasomotor symptoms: Sweating, hot flushes, palpitations	1. Genital atrophy: Loss of superficial keratinised cells, thinning of the vaginal mucosa, reduced secretions from the glands, and increase in vaginal pH 2. Pelvic organ prolapse 3. Reduction in collagen support and atrophy: Increased vulnerability to trauma and infection, skin changes, and easy bruising 4. Urodynamic changes: Stress incontinence, urgency, and an increased frequency of urination	Cardiovascular effects Dementia *Osteoporosis*: Due to oestrogen deficiency and affects the trabecular bone

APPENDIX

CHAPTER 29
Mnemonics

ANATOMY

1. **Layers of the scrotum (**S**ome** D**amn** E**nglishmen** C**alled** I**t** T**he** T**estis)**

   - **S**kin
   - **D**artos
   - **E**xternal spermatic fascia
   - **C**remaster muscle
   - **I**nternal spermatic fascia
   - **T**unica vaginalis
   - **T**estis

2. **Borders of the femoral triangle (shaped like a SAIL)**
   - **S**artorius
   - **A**dductor longus
   - **I**nguinal **L**igament

3. **Level of diaphragmatic apertures**

   - Vena cava = 8 letters = T8
   - Oesophagus = 10 letters = T10
   - Aortic hiatus = 12 letters = T12

4. **Nerve root supply of deep tendon reflexes (one, two – buckle my shoe, three, four – kick the door, five, six – pick up sticks, seven, eight – shut the gate)**

   - S1, S2 – ankle jerk
   - L3, L4 – knee jerk
   - C5, C6 – biceps and brachioradialis
   - C7, C8 – triceps

7. Relations of ureter and uterine artery/ vas deferens (water runs under the bridge)

Ureter (water) runs posteriorly to uterine artery/ vas deferens (bridge)

8. Axillary artery branches (Some Times Life Seems A Pain)

- **S**uperior thoracic
- **T**horacoacromiol
- **L**ateral thoracic
- **S**ubscapular
- **A**nterior circumflex humeral
- **P**osterior circumflex humeral

9. Femoral triangle: arrangement of contents (NAVEL)

From lateral hip towards medial **navel**:
- **N**erve (directly behind sheath)
- **A**rtery (within sheath)
- **V**ein (within sheath)
- **E**mpty space (between vein and lymph)
- **L**ymphatics (with deep inguinal node)

10. Contents of the tarsal tunnel

(From anterior to posterior Tom, Dick And Very Nervous Harry)

- **T**ibialis posterior
- flexor **D**igitorum longus
- **A**rtery (posterior tibial)
- **V**ein (posterior tibial)
- **N**erve (tibial)
- Flexor **H**allucis longus

11. Relations of femoral nerve, artery and vein (from lateral to medial NAVY)

MNEMONICS

- Nerve
- Artery
- Vein
- LYmphatics (femoral canal)

12. Thoracoacromial artery branches (ABCD)
- **A**cromial
- **B**reast (pectoral)
- **C**lavicular
- **D**eltoid

13. Abdominal muscles (Spare TIRE around their abdomen)
- **T**ransversus abdominis
- **I**nternal abdominal oblique
- **R**ectus abdominis
- **E**xternal abdominal oblique

14. Elbow: muscles that flex it
(Three **B**'s **B**end the elbow)

- **B**rachialis
- **B**iceps
- **B**rachioradialis

15. Wrist bones (She Looks Too Pretty, Try To Catch Her)
- **S**caphoid
- **L**unate
- **T**riquetrum
- **P**isiform
- **T**rapezium
- **T**rapezoid
- **C**apitate
- **H**amate

16. Attachments of pectoralis major, teres major and latissimus dorsi to the bicipital groove **(a lady between two majors)**
- Pectoralis **major** attaches laterally

- Teres **major** attaches medially
- **Latissimus dorsi** ('lady') attaches to the floor **in between**

17. Inguinal canal: walls (MALT: 2M, 2A, 2L, 2T1)

   Starting from superior, moving around in order to posterior:
   - Superior wall (roof): 2 **M**uscles:
     - Internal oblique **M**uscle
     - Transverse abdominus **M**uscle
   - Anterior wall: 2 **A**poneuroses:
     - **A**poneurosis of external oblique
     - **A**poneurosis of internal oblique
   - Lower wall (floor): 2 **L**igaments:
     - Inguinal **L**igament
     - Lacunar **L**igament
   - Posterior wall: 2**T**s:
     - **T**ransversalis fascia
     - Conjoint **T**endon

18. Broad ligament: contents (BROAD)
    - **B**undle (ovarian neurovascular bundle)
    - **R**ound ligament
    - **O**varian ligament
    - **A**rtefacts (vestigial structures)
    - **D**uct (oviduct)

PHYSIOLOGY

1. **Osteoblast versus osteoclast**

   - Osteo**B**last **B**uilds bone.
   - Osteo**C**last **C**onsumes (breakdown) bone.

2. **Alkalosis vs. acidosis: directions of pH and HCO₃ (ROME)**

   - **R**espiratory= **O**pposite:

- pH is high, PCO_2 is down (Alkalosis)
- pH is low, PCO_2 is up (Acidosis)
- Metabolic= Equal:
  - pH is high, HCO_3 is high (Alkalosis)
  - pH is low, HCO_3 is low (Acidosis)

3. **Prolactin and oxytocin: functions**
   - **PRO**lactin stimulates the mammary glands to **PRO**duce milk.
   - **O**xytocin stimulates the mammary glands to **O**oze (release) milk.

4. **Pituitary hormones (FLAGTOP)**
   - **F**ollicle stimulating hormone
   - **L**utinizing hormone
   - **A**drenocorticotropin hormone
   - **G**rowth hormone
   - **T**hyroid stimulating hormone
   - **O**xytocin
   - **P**rolactin

5. **Erythropoiesis stages (Powerful Businesses Pollute Our Reeling Environment)**
   - Proerythroblast
   - Basophilic erythroblast
   - Polychromatic erythroblast
   - Orthochromatophilic erythroblast
   - Reticulocyte
   - Erythrocyte

6. **Hyperthyroidism: signs and symptoms (THYROIDISM)**
   - **T**remor
   - **H**eart rate increases
   - **Y**awning (fatigability)
   - **R**estlessness
   - **O**ligomenorrhea & amenorrhea

- o Intolerance to heat
- o **D**iarrhea
- o **I**rritability
- o **S**weating
- o **M**usle wasting & weight loss

7. **LH vs FSH: function in male**

    - o **LH: L**eydig cells stimulated to produce testosterone.
    - o **FSH: S**permatogenesis stimulated.

8. **Hb-oxygen dissociation curve shifts: effect, location**
    - o **L**eft shift: causes **L**oading of O_2 in **L**ungs.
    - o **R**ight shift: causes **R**elease of O_2 from Hb.

9. **Carotid sinus vs. carotid body function**

    - o carotid **SinuS**: measures pre**SS**ure.
    - o carotid b**O**dy measures **O2**.

10. **Adrenal gland: functions (ACTH)**

    - o **A**drenergic functions
    - o **C**atabolism of proteins/**C**arbohydrate metabolism
    - o **T** cell immunomodulation
    - o **H**yper/**H**ypotension (blood pressure control)

11. **Fluid compartments: volumes (12345)**

    - o **12** liters of interstitial fluid
    - o **3** liters plasma volume and **30** liters inside cells
    - o **45** liters total body water

12. **Gut intrinsic innervation: myenteric plexus vs. submucosal plexus function**

- **Myenteric**: **M**otility.
- **Submucosal**: **S**ecretion and blood flow.

13. Glucagon: actions (LKG2)

- **L**ipolysis
- **K**etogenesis
- **G**lycogenolysis
- **G**luconeogenesis

14. Muscle sarcomere: H line vs. Z disc location [HAZI (Hazy)]

- **H** line is in **A**-band.
- **Z** disc is in the **I** band.

15. Alkalosis: metabolic changes in alkalosis

(Al-K-loss, Al-Ca-loss)

There is loss of K+ (hypokalemia) and Ca++ (hypocalcemia) in state of alkalosis.

16. Haematology: key numbers

3 and 4 are key numbers in haematology:

1.34 cm^3 of oxygen is carried by a gram of hemoglobin.
There's 3.4mg of iron in each gram of hemoglobin.
There's an average of 3.4 lobes per neutrophil.
There's 34mg bilirubin from each gram of hemoglobin.

17. Wernicke's and Broca's areas (BEWaRe)
- **B**roca's defect—**E**xpressive aphasia
- **W**ernicke's defect—**R**eceptive aphasia

BIOCHEMISTRY

1. Citric acid cycle components

(Oh! Can I Keep Some Succinate For Myself?)

- **O**xaloacetate
- **C**itrate
- **I**socitrate
- **K**etoglutanate
- **S**uccinyl CoA
- **Succinate**
- **F**umarate
- **M**alate

2. B vitamin names
(**T**he **R**hythm **N**early **P**roved **C**ontagious)

In increasing order:
- **T**hiamine (B1)
- **R**iboflavin (B2)
- **N**iacin (B3)
- **P**yridoxine (B6)
- **C**obalamin (B12)

3. Essential amino acids (**PVT. TIM HALL** never **t**ires)

1. **P**he (phenylalanine)
2. **V**al (valine)
3. **T**hr (threonine)
4. **T**rp (tryptophan)
5. **I**le (isoleucine)
6. **M**et (methionine)
7. **H**is (histidine)
8. **L**ue (leucine)
9. **L**ys (lysine)

"Never tires": T is not Tyr, but is both Thr and Trp.

4. **Branched chain amino acids (LEVIS)**

   - **LE**ucine
   - **V**aline
   - **IS**oleucine

5. **Fasting state: branched-chain amino acids used by skeletal muscles** (Muscles **LIV**e fast)

   - **L**eucine
   - **I**soleucine
   - **V**aline

6. **Causes of metabolic acidosis with raised anion gap (MUDPILES)**
   - **M**ethanol
   - **U**raemia
   - **D**iabetic ketoacidosis (and alcoholic/starvation ketoacidosis)
   - **P**ropylene glycol
   - **I**soniazid
   - **L**actate
   - **E**thylene glycol
   - **S**alicylates

7. **Folate deficiency: causes (A FOLIC DROP)**

   - **A**lcoholism
   - **F**olic acid antagonists
   - **O**ral contraceptives
   - **L**ow dietary intake
   - **I**nfection with Giardia
   - **C**eliac sprue
   - **D**ilatin (phenytoin)
   - **R**elative folate deficiency
   - **O**ld
   - **P**regnancy

8. **Glycogen storage: names of types I through VI** (**V**iagra **P**ills **C**ause **A** **M**ajor **H**eadache for **T**im)

    o GSD I: **V**on Gierke's
    o GSD II: **P**ompe's
    o GSD III: **C**ori's
    o GSD IV: **A**nderson's
    o GSD V: **M**cArdle's
    o GSD VI: **H**er's
    o GSD VII: **T**auri's

9. **G6PD deficiency: oxidant drugs inducing hemolytic anemia (AAA)**

    o **A**ntibiotic (eg: sufamethoxazole)
    o **A**ntimalarial (eg: primaquine)
    o **A**ntipyretics (eg: acetanilid, but not aspirin or acetaminophen)

10. **Glycolysis steps**
(**G**oodness **G**racious, **F**ather **F**ranklin **D**id **G**o **B**y **P**icking **P**umpkins (to) **Pr**e**p**are **P**ie**s**)

    o **G**lucose
    o **G**lucose-6-P
    o **F**ructose-6-P
    o **F**ructose-1,6-diP
    o **D**ihydroxyacetone-P
    o **G**lyceraldehyde-P
    o 1,3-**Bi**phosphoglycerate
    o 3-**P**hosphoglycerate
    o 2-**P**hosphoglycerate (to)
    o Phosphoenolpyruvate [**PEP**]
    o **P**yruvate

"**Did**", "**By**" and "**Pies**" tell you the first part of those three: di-, bi-, and py-.
"**PrEP**are" tells location of PEP in the process.

MNEMONICS

11. Hypervitaminosis A: signs and symptoms (Increased Vitamin A makes you **HARD**)

- **H**eadache/ **H**epatomegaly
- **A**norexia/ **A**lopecia
- **R**eally painful bones
- **D**ry skin/ **D**rowsiness

12. Cell division (**P**eople **M**eet **A**nd **T**alk)
- **P**rophase
- **M**etaphase
- **A**naphase
- **T**elophase

13. Vitamin B3 (niacin, nicotinic acid) deficiency: pellagra (The 3 **D**'s of pellagra)

- **D**ermatitis
- **D**iarrhea
- **D**ementia

14. Vitamins: which are fat soluble (KADE)

- Vitamin **K**
- Vitamin **A**
- Vitamin **D**
- Vitamin **E**

15. Fabry's disease (FABRY'S)

- **F**oam cells found in glomeruli and tubules/**F**ebrile episodes
- **A**lpha galactosidase A deficiency/**A**ngiokeratomas
- **B**urning pain in extremities/**B**UN increased in serum/**B**oys
- **R**enal failure
- **Y**X genotype (male, X linked recessive)
- **S**phingolipidoses

16. **Hemoglobin binding curve: causes of shift to right (CADET, face right!)**

    - CO_2
    - **A**cid
    - 2,3-**D**PG
    - **E**xercise
    - **T**emperature

17. **Porphyrias: acute intermittent porphyria symptoms** (5 P's)

    - **P**ain in abdomen
    - **P**olyneuropathy
    - **P**sychologial abnormalities
    - **P**ink coloured urine
    - **P**recipitated by drugs (e.g. barbiturates, oral contraceptives, sulpha drugs)

18. **Sickle cell anemia: mutation**

    (Hb**S** isn't **V**ery **G**ood)

At **S**ixth position of HB beta chain, **V**aline is present instead of **G**lutamic acid.

19. **Adrenaline mechanism (ABC of Adrenaline)**

Adrenaline --> activates **B**eta receptors --> increases **C**yclic AMP

20. **BUN: creatinine elevation: causes (ABCD)**
    - **A**zotremia (pre-renal)
    - **B**leeding (GI)
    - **C**atabolic status
    - **D**iet (high protein parenteral nutrition)

21. **Insulin: function**

INsulIN stimulates **2** things to go **IN 2** cells: Potassium and Glucose.

22. DNA bond strength (nucleotides) (Crazy Glue)

Strongest bonds are between **C**ytosine and **G**uanine, strong like **C**razy **G**lue (3 H-bonds), whereas the A=T only have 2 H-bonds. (This fact is significant in relation to the DNA replication, because the weaker A=T will be the site where RNA primer makes the initial break.)

23. Enzyme kinetics: competitive vs. non-competitive inhibition

- With **K**ompetitive inhibition: **K**m increases; no change in Vmax.
- With **N**on-kompetitive inhibition: **N**o change in **K**m; **V**max decreases.

PATHOLOGY

1. Gallstones: risk factors (5 F's)

- Fat
- Female
- Family history
- Fertile
- Forty

2. Carcinoid syndrome: components (CARCinoid)

- **C**utaneous flushing
- **A**sthmatic wheezing
- **R**ight sided valvular heart lesions
- **C**ramping and diarrhea

3. Hematuria: urethral causes (NUTS)
- **N**eoplasm
- **U**rethritis

- Tumour
- Stone

4. Hepatomegaly: 3 common causes, 3 rarer causes

(Common are 3 C's)
- Cirrhosis
- Carcinoma
- Cardiac failure

(Rarer are 3 C's)

- Cholestasis
- Cysts
- Cellular infiltration

5. Ulcerative colitis: features (ULCERATIONS)

- Ulcers
- Large intestine
- Carcinoma [risk]
- Extraintestinal manifestations
- Remnants of old ulcers [pseudopolyps]
- Abscesses in crypts
- Toxic megacolon [risk]
- Inflamed, red, granular mucosa
- Originates at rectum
- Neutrophil invasion
- Stools bloody

6. Portal hypertension: features (ABCDE)

- Ascites
- Bleeding (haematemesis, piles)
- Caput medusa
- Diminished liver
- Enlarged spleen

7. Cushing syndrome (CUSHING)

- **C**entral obesity/ Cervical fat pads/ Collagen fiber weakness/ Comedones (acne)
- **U**rinary free corisol and glucose increase
- **S**triae/ Suppressed immunity
- **H**ypercortisolism/ Hypertension/ Hyperglycemia/ Hirsutism
- **I**atrogenic (Increased administration of corticosteroids)
- **N**oniatrogenic (Neoplasms)
- **G**lucose intolerance/ Growth retardation

8. Duchenne vs. Becker Muscular Dystrophy

- Duchenne Muscular Dystrophy (DMD): Doesn't Make Dystrophin.
- Becker Muscular Dystrophy (BMD): Badly Made Dystrophin (due to mutations in the dystrophin gene resulting in a truncated protein).

9. Anemia (normocytic): causes (ABCD)

- **A**cute blood loss
- **B**one marrow failure
- **C**hronic disease
- **D**estruction (hemolysis)

10. Hypercalcemia: Symptoms (Bones, Stones, Groans, Moans)

- **Bones**-Pain in bones
- **Stones**-Renal
- **Groans**-Pain
- **Moans**-Psychic Moans, Confused State

11. Blood disorders: commoner sex

HE (male) gets:
- **HE**mophilia (X-linked)

- HEinz bodies (G6PD deficiency, causing HEmolytic anemia: X-linked)
- HEmochromatosis (male predominance)
- HEart attacks (male predominance)
- HEnoch-Schonlein purpura (male predominance)

SHE (female) gets:
- SHEehan's syndrome

12. Pulmonary Embolism Risk Factors (Tom Schrepfer)

- **T**rauma
- **O**besity
- **M**alignancy
- **S**urgery
- **C**ardiac dis
- **H**ospitalization
- **R**est(bed ridden)
- **E**lderly
- **P**ast history
- **F**racture
- **E**strogen(pregnancy, postpartum)
- **R**oad trip

13. Fat embolism: findings (Fat, Bat, Fract)
- **Fat** in urine, sputum
- **Bat**-wing (lung x-ray)
- **Fract**ure history: Fracture of **FEM**ur causes Fat **EM**boli.

14. Deep venous thrombosis: diagnosis (DVT)

- **D**ilated superficial veins/ **D**iscoloration/ **D**oppler ultrasound
- **V**enography is gold standard
- **T**enderness of **T**high and calf

15. Disseminated Intravascular Cogulation: causes (DIC)

- **D**elivery **TEAR** (obstetric complications)
- **I**nfections (gram negative)/ **I**mmunological

- Cancer (prostate, pancreas, lung, stomach)

Obstretrical complications are **(TEAR)**
- **T**oxemia of pregnancy
- **E**mboli (amniotic)
- **A**brutio placentae
- **R**etained fetal products

16. **Wernick-Korsakov Syndrome (CAN of beer)**

- **C**onfusion
- **A**taxia
- **N**ystagmus

17. **Nephrotic syndrome: hallmark findings (Protein LEAC)**

- **Protein**uria (In nephrotic nsyndrome, the **proteins leak** out)
- **L**ipid levels increase
- **E**dema
- **A**lbumin levels reduce
- **C**holesterol levels increase

18. **Megaloblastic anemia: vitamin B12 deficiency vs. folate deficiency**

Vitamin **B**12 deficiency also affects **B**rain (optic neuropathy, subacute combined degeneration, paresthesia).

Folate deficiency is not associated with neurological symptoms.

MICROBIOLOGY

1. **Flavivirus: Diseases caused (WeeDs of JOY)**
   - **W**est nile fever
   - **D**engue
   - **J**apanese B encephaliis

- Omsk hemorrhagic fever (OHF)
- Yellow fever

2. **Picorna viridae: members (PEECoRnA)** (Picorna is pronounced "pee-corna")

    - **P**oliovirus
    - **E**chovirus
    - **E**nterovirus
    - **Co**ronavirus
    - **R**hinovirus
    - Hepatitis **A**

3. **Vibrio: motility (Vibrio Vibrates)**
    - Vibrio is a genus of actively motile bacteria.

4. **Vibrio cholerae: biochemical reactions which help to differentiate vibrio cholera (COINS)**

    - **C**atalase +ve
    - **O**xidase +ve
    - **I**ndole +ve
    - **N**itrates reduced to nitrites
    - **S**ucrose fermentation

5. **Endocarditis: lab results** (High Tech Lab Results Point At Endocarditis)

    - **H**ematuria
    - **T**hrombocytopenia
    - **L**eukocytosis, -penia
    - **R**ed blood cell casts
    - **P**roteinuria
    - **A**nemia
    - **E**levated ESR

6. **Catalase positive organism (SPACE)**

    - **S**taphylococcus aureus

- Pseudomonas
- Aspergillus
- Candida
- Enterobacter

7. UTI-causing microorganisms (KEEPS)

- Klebsiella
- Enterococcus faecalis/ Enterobacter cloacae
- E. coli
- Pseudomonas aeroginosa/ Proteus mirabilis
- Staphylococcus saprophyticcus/ Serratia marcescens

8. Urease positive organisms (PUNCH)

- Proteus (leads to alkaline urine)
- Ureaplasma (renal calculi)
- Nocardia
- Cryptoccocus (the fungus)
- Helicobacter pylori

9. Chlamydia: elementary vs. initial body location
- Elementary: Extracellular
- Initial: Intracellular

10. Common cold: viral causes (acute infectious rhinitis, coryza is PRIMArily caused by)

- Paramyxoviruses
- Rhinoviruses
- Influenza viruses
- Myxoviruses
- Adenoviruses

11. Placenta-crossing organisms/ antenatal Infections (STARCH)

- Syphilis
- Toxoplasmosis

- AIDS (HIV)
- Rubella
- CMV
- Herpes/Hepatitis

12. Neisseria: Fermentation of N. gonorrhoeae vs. N. meningitidis

- **G**onorrhoeae: **G**lucose fermenter only.
- **M**enin**G**itidis: **M**altose and **G**lucose fermenter.

Maltose fermentation is a classical test which helps distinguish the various Neisseria types.

13. Staphylococcus aureus: Diseases caused (SOFT PAINS)

- **S**kin infections
- **O**steomyelitis
- **F**ood poisoning
- **T**oxic shock syndrome
- **P**neumonia
- **A**cute endocarditis
- **I**nfective arthritis
- **N**ecrotizing fasciitis
- **S**epsis

14. Streptococci: classification by hemolytic ability

- **Ga**mma: **Ga**rbage (no hemolytic activity).
- **Al**pha: **Al**most (almost lyse, but incomplete).
- **Be**ta: **Be**st (complete lysis).

15. Mycobacterium tuberculosis: culture identification

(Rough, Tough, Buff)
- **Rough**: colony isn't smooth but rough like breadcrumbs.
- **Tough**: colony stuck to plate well, and tough to remove.
- **Buff**: buff is a color, a cream/coffee shade.

16. Streptococcus pyogenes: Diseases caused (NIPPLES)

- Necrotising fasciitis and myositis
- Impetigo
- Pharyngitis
- Pneumonia
- Lymphangitis
- Erysipelas and cellulitis
- Scarlet fever/ Streptococcal TSS

17. Teratogens: placenta-crossing organisms (TORCHES)

- Toxoplasma
- Others (parvo, listeria)
- Rubella
- CMV
- Herpes simplex, Herpes zoster (varicella), Hepatitis B,C,E, HIV
- Enteroviruses
- Syphilis

18. Trichomaniasis: features (5 F's)
- Flagella
- Frothy discharge
- Fishy odor (sometimes)
- Fornication (STD)
- Flagyl (metronidazole) Rx

IMMUNOLOGY

1. **MHC I vs. II: T cell interaction**
   (The "=8" equation: $2 \times 4 = 8$, and $1 \times 8 = 8$
   MHC **II** goes with CD**4**.
   MHC **I** goes with CD**8**.

2. **Acute inflammation features (SLIPR)**
   - Swelling
   - Loss of function
   - Increased heat

- Pain
- Redness

3. **Celiac sprue features (CELIAC)**

   - **C**ell-mediated autoimmune disease
   - **E**uropean descent
   - **L**ymphocytes in **L**amina propria/ **L**ymphoma risk
   - **I**ntolerance of gluten (wheat)
   - **A**trophy of villi in small intestine/ **A**bnormal D-xylose test (Atrophied villi cause less absorption, so diarrhea, weight loss, less energy)
   - **C**hildhood presentation

4. **HLA-DR genetic predisposition immune disease examples (HLA-DR)**

   - **H**ashimoto's disease
   - **L**eukemia/ **L**upus
   - **A**utoimmune adrenalitis/**A**nemia (pernicious)
   - **D**iabetes insipidous
   - **R**heumatoid arthritis

5. **DiGeorge Syndrome: features (**The disease of **T**'s)

   - **T**hird and 4th pharyngeal pouch absent.
   - **T**wenty-**T**wo chromosome (deletion of a small segment)
   - **T**-cells absent
   - **T**etany: Hypocalcemia

6. **Goodpasture's Syndrome components**
   - **G**ood**P**asture is **G**lomerulonephritis and **P**nuemonitits.
   - Caused by autoantibodies attacking **G**lomerular and **P**ulmonary basement membranes.

7. Macrophages differentiate into specialized forms in different tissues **(KOMA)**
- **K**upffer cells (liver)
- **O**steoclasts (bone)

- Microglia (CNS)
- Alveolar macrophages (lung)

8. **Immunoglobulins: which crosses the placenta**
   Ig**G** crosses the placenta during **G**estation.

9. **SLE (Systemic Lupus Erythematosus) diagnosis (ARA criteria) (DAMP AS RHINO)**
- **D**iscoid rash
- **A**NA (+)
- **M**alar rash
- **P**hotosensitivity
- **A**rthritis
- **S**erositis (pleural, pericardial)
- **R**enal involvement
- **H**ematologic abnormality
- **I**mmunologic abnormality
- **N**eurologic abnormality (seizures, psychosis)
- **O**ral / nasal ulcer

10. **Sjogren syndrome: morphology** (**J**og through the **MAPLES**)
Sj**og**ren is:
- **M**outh dry
- **A**rthritis
- **P**arotid enlarged
- **L**ymphoma
- **E**yes dry
- **S**icca (primary) or **S**econdary

11. **Microcytic anemia: causes (Find Those Small Cells)**

- **F**e deficiency
- **T**halassemia
- **S**ideroblastic
- **C**hronic disease

EMBRYOLOGY

1. 2nd, 3rd and 4th weeks of development:

- Week 2: Bilaminar germ disc
- Week 3: Trilaminar germ disc
- Week 4: Appearance of 4 limbs

2. Major Neural Crest Derivatives (GAMES)

- **G**lial cells of peripheral ganglia
- **A**rachnoid and Pia Sheath
- **M**elanocytes
- **E**nteric ganglia
- **S**chwann cells

3. Woffian duct (mesonephric duct) derivatives (Gardener's SEED)

- Female: **Gartner's** duct, cyst
- Male:
    - **S**eminal vesicles
    - **E**pididymis
    - **E**jaculatory duct
    - **D**uctus deferens

4. Foregut derivatives (Little Embryo People Do Like Swaying and Playing Games)

- Lungs
- Esophagus
- Pancreas
- Duodenum (proximal)
- Liver
- Stomach
- Pancreas
- Gall bladder

5. Lung Development Phases (Every Premature Child Takes Air)

MNEMONICS

- Embryonic period
- Pseudoglandular period
- Canalicular period
- Terminal sac period
- Alveolar period

6. **Branchial apparatus (CAP** covers from outside to inside.)

   - **C** for **C**lefts : derived from ectoderm
   - **A** for **A**rches : derived from mesoderm and neural crest
   - **P** for **P**ouches : derived from endoderm

7. **Substances which cross placenta (WANT My HotDog)**

   - **W**astes
   - **A**ntibodies
   - **N**utrients
   - **T**eratogens
   - **M**icroorganism
   - **H**ormone/HIV
   - **D**rugs

8. **Cartilage derivatives of 2nd branchial arch: (5 "S")**

   - **S**tapes
   - **S**tyloid process
   - **S**tylohyoid ligament
   - **S**maller (lesser) cornu of hyoid
   - **S**uperior part of body of hyoid

9. **Derivatives of Pharyngeal Pouches: (1A, 2P, 3 TIP, 4 SPUB)**

   - **1A** (1st Pharyngeal Pouch – **A**uditory)
     Epithelial lining of Auditory tube, middle ear cavity and mastoid antrum
   - **2P** (2nd Pharyngeal Pouch – **P**alatine)
     Epithelial lining of crypts of Palatine tonsil

- **3 TIP** (3rd Pharyngeal Pouch – **T**hymus and **I**nferior **P**arathyroid gland)
- **4 SPUB** (4th Pharyngeal Pouch – **S**uperior **P**arathyroid gland and **U**ltimobranchial **B**ody)

10. Potter syndrome: features (POTTER)
- **P**ulmonary hypoplasia
- **O**ligohydrominios
- **T**wisted skin (wrinkly skin)
- **T**wisted face (Potter facies)
- **E**xtremities defects
- **R**enal agenesis (bilateral)

11. Mesoderm components (MESODERM)

- **M**esothelium (peritoneal, pleural, pericardial)/ **M**uscle (striated, smooth, cardiac)
- **E**mbryologic **S**pleen/ **S**oft tissue/ **S**erous linings/ **S**arcoma/ **S**omite
- **O**sseous tissue/ **O**uter layer of suprarenal gland (cortex)/ **O**varies
- **D**ura/ **D**ucts of genitalia
- **E**ndothelium
- **R**enal **M**icroglia
- **M**esenchyme/ **M**ale gonad

12. Teratogenesis: when it occurs

- **TE**ratogenesis is most likely during organogenesis--between the: **T**hird and **E**ighth weeks of gestation.

13. Tetrology of Fallot (Don't **DROP** the baby)

- **D**efect (VSD)
- **R**ight ventricular hypertrophy
- **O**verriding aorta
- **P**ulmonary stenosis

GENETICS

1. **Achrondroplasia dwarfism: inheritance pattern**
   - Achondroplasia Dwarfism is Autosomal Dominant.

2. **Down syndrome features (My CHILD HAS PROBLEM!)**

   - Congenital heart disease/ Cataracts
   - Hypotonia / Hypothyroidism
   - Increased gap between 1st and 2nd toe
   - Leukemia risk x 2/ Lung problem
   - Duodenal atresia / Delayed development
   - Hirshsprung's disease / Hearing loss /
   - Alzheimer's disease / Atlantoaxial instability
   - Squint/ Short neck /Short fifth finger (with hypoplasia of the middle phalanx)
   - Protruding tongue/ Palm crease
   - Round face/ Rolling eye (nystagmus)
   - Occiput flat/ Oblique eye fissure
   - Brushfield spot/ Brachycephaly
   - Low nasal bridge/ Language problem
   - Epicanthic fold/ Ear folded
   - Mental retardation/ Myoclonus

3. **Tay Sach's features (SACHS)**
   - Spot in macula
   - Ashkenazic Jews
   - CNS degeneration
   - Hexosaminidase A deficiency
   - Storage disease

   Extra details with **TAY**:
   - Testing recommended
   - Autosomal recessive/ Amaurosis
   - Young death (<4 yrs)

4. **Blots: function of Southern vs. Northern vs. Western (SN0W DR0P)**

Match up the letter of the 1st word (**SN0W**) with the letter of 2nd word (**DR0P**).
- **S**outhern=**D**NA
- **N**orthern=**R**NA
- **Z**ero (none)=**E**astern
- **W**estern=**P**rotein

The 0's in snow drop are zeros, since there is no Eastern blot.

5. **Cell cycle stages (Go Sally Go! Meet Children)**

- **G**1 phase (Growth phase 1)
- **S** phase (DNA Synthesis)
- **G**2 phase (Growth phase 2)
- **M** phase (Mitosis)
- **C** phase (Cytokinesis)

6. **Chromosome 15 diseases (**Chromosome 15 has its own **MAP)**
- **M**arfan syndrome
- **A**ngelman syndrome
- **P**rader-Willi syndrome

7. **Down syndrome pathology (DOWN)**

- **D**ecreased alpha-fetoprotein and unconjugated estriol (maternal)
- **O**ne extra chromosome twenty-one
- **W**omen of advanced age
- **N**ondisjunction during maternal meiosis

8. **Hurler syndrome features (HURLER'S)**

- **H**eptosplenomegaly
- **U**gly facies
- **R**ecessive (AR inheritance)
- **L**-iduronidase deficiency (alpha)
- **E**yes clouded

- o **R**etarded
- o **S**hort/ **S**tubby fingers

9. Marfan syndrome features (MARFAN'S)

- o **M**itral valve prolapse
- o **A**ortic **A**neurysm
- o **R**etinal detachment
- o **F**ibrillin (mutations of this gene)
- o **A**rachnodactyly
- o **N**egative **N**itroprusside test (differentiates from homocystinuria)
- o **S**ubluxated lens

10. Nucleotides: class having the single ring

(Pyrimadines are **CUT** from purines)
- o Pyrimidines are:
    - **C**ytosine
    - **U**racil
    - **T**hiamine
- o They are **cut** from purines so the pyrimadines must be smaller (one ring).

11. Nucleotides: double vs. triple bonded basepairs

[**TU** bonds (two bonds)]

- o **T**-A and **U**-A have **Two** bonds.
- o G-C therefore has the three bonds

12. Features of Fragile X syndrome (Rule of M's)

- o **M**ale
- o **M**acro-orchidism
- o **M**ental retardation
- o **M**axillary excess (long face)
- o **M**uscle tone decrease
- o **M**ovements stereotyped

- o Mutation in FMR1 gene
- o Multiple CGG repeats
- o Mothers (females) are obligatory carriers

13. **Nucleotides: which are purines**

(Pure Silver)
Chemical formula of **Pur**e silver is **Ag**.
Therefore, **Pur**ines are **A**denine and **G**uanine.

EPIDEMEIOLOGY

1. **Prevalence of disease (PID)**
   Prevalence = Incidence x Duration
2. **Sensitivity and Specificity**
   - o se**N**sitivity of a test: related to the rate of false **N**egatives **(N**o **N**on-**N**egatives)
   - o s**P**ecificity of a test: related to the rate of false **P**ositives. (**P**uny **P**suedo-**P**ositives)

3. **Informed consent: requirements** (Sign this **DOC** before we can start)

   - o **D**iscussion
   - o **O**btain agreement
   - o **C**oercion-free

4. **Informed consent:** Exceptions (**WIPE**)

   - o **W**aiver
   - o **I**ncompetent
   - o **P**rivilege (therapeutic privilege)
   - o **E**mergency

5. **Error: type I (alpha) vs. type II (beta)**

Type I (Alpha) Error: "There Is An Effect" where in reality there is none.

MNEMONICS

6. **Polio Virus Strains (OPV)**

   - type 1 : **O** = Outbreaks of paralytic polio
   - type 2 : **P** = Potent antigenic strain
   - type 3 : **V** = Vaccine associated polio

7. **Passively immunized diseases with antisera** (DetecTive BRG)

   - **D**iptheria
   - **T**etanus
   - **B**otulism
   - **R**abies
   - **G**as gangrene

8. **Live attenuated vaccines** (ROME Is My Best Place To go Yet)

   - **R**ubella
   - **O**ral polio vaccine (OPV)
   - **M**easles
   - **E**pidemic typhus
   - **I**nfluenza
   - **M**umps
   - **B**CG
   - **P**lague
   - **T**yphoid oral vaccine
   - **Y**ellow fever

9. **Notifiable Diseases** (Yellow CuP)
   - **Y**ellow fever
   - **C**holera
   - **P**lague

PHARMACOLOGY

1. **Antiarrhythmics: class III members (BIAS)**

- Bretylium
- Ibutilide
- Amiodarone
- Sotalol

2. **Hepatic necrosis: drugs causing focal to massive necrosis (Very Angry Hepatocytes):**
- Valproic acid
- Acetaminophen
- Halothane

3. **Adrenoceptors: vasomotor function of alpha vs. beta (ABCD)**
- Alpha = Constrict
- Beta = Dilate

4. **Beta-blockers: main contraindications (ABCDE)**
- Asthma
- Block (heart block)
- COPD
- Diabetes mellitus
- Electrolyte abnormality (hyperkalemia)

5. **Captopril (an ACE inhibitor): side effects (CAPTOPRIL)**

- Cough
- Angioedema/ Agranulocystosis
- Proteinuria/ Potassium excess
- Taste changes
- Orthostatic hypotension
- Pregnancy contraindication/ Pancreatitis/ Pressure drop (first dose hypertension)
- Renal failure (and renal artery stenosis contraindication)/ Rash
- Indomethacin inhibition
- Leukopenia/ Liver toxicity

6. **Beta-blockers: nonselective beta-blockers (Tim Places His Name Plate)**

- Timolol
- Pindolol
- Hismolol
- Naldolol
- Propranolol

14. **Fetal alcohol syndrome (FAS)**

- **F**acial hypoplasia and **F**orebrain malformation
- **A**ttention deficit disorder and **A**ltered joints
- **S**hort stature, **S**eptal defects and **S**mall I.Q

15. **Cardioselectives Beta Blockers** (**B**eta Blockers **A**cting **E**xclusively **A**t **M**yocardium)

- **B**etaxolol
- **A**cebutolol
- **E**smolol
- **A**tenolol
- **M**etoprolol

14. Ventricular Tachycardia: Rx **(LAMB)**

- **L**idocaine
- **A**miodarone
- **M**exiltine
- **B**eta blocker

7. **Patent ductus arteriosus: treatment** (Come **In** and **Close** the door)
- **IN**domethacin is used to **Close** PDA.

8. **Thrombolytic agents (USA)**

- **U**rokinase
- **S**treptokinase
- **A**lteplase (tPA)

9. **K+ increasing agents (K-BANK)**

- K-sparing diuretic
- Beta blocker
- ACE Inhibitors
- NSAID
- K supplement

10. Gynaecomastia-causing drugs (DISCOS)

- **D**igoxin
- **I**soniazid
- **S**pironolactone
- **C**imetidine
- **O**estrogens
- **S**tilboestrol

11. Propythiouracil (PTU): mechanism (It inhibits PTU):
- **P**eroxidase/ **P**eripheral deiodination
- **T**yrosine iodination
- **U**nion (coupling)

12. Lupus: drugs inducing it (HIP)

- **H**ydralazine
- **I**NH
- **P**rocanimide

13. Steroids: side effects (BECLOMETHASONE)
- **B**uffalo hump
- **E**asy bruising
- **C**ataracts
- **L**arger appetite
- **O**besity
- **M**oonface
- **E**uphoria
- **T**hin arms & legs
- **H**ypertension/ **H**yperglycaemia
- **A**vascular necrosis of femoral head
- **S**kin thinning

- o Osteoporosis
- o Negative nitrogen balance
- o Emotional liability

14. Diuretics (thiazides) indications (CHIC)
- o CHF
- o Hypertension
- o Insipidus (diabetes)
- o Calcium calculi

15. Nitrofurantoin: major side effects (NitroFurAntoin)

- o Neuropathy (peripheral neuropathy)
- o Fibrosis (pulmonary fibrosis)
- o Anemia (hemolytic anemia)

16. Tetracycline: teratogenicity

- o **TE**tracycline is a
- o **TE**ratogen that causes staining of
- o **TE**eth in the newborn.

17. SIADH-inducing drugs (ABCD)

- o **A**nalgesics: opioids, NSAIDs
- o **B**arbiturates
- o **C**yclophosphamide/ **C**hlorpromazine/ **C**arbamazepine
- o **D**iuretic (thiazide)

18. Osmotic diuretics: members (GUM)
- o Glycerol
- o Urea
- o Mannitol

19. Sulfonamide: major side effects (4S)

- o Steven-Johnson syndrome
- o Skin rash
- o Solubility low (causes crystalluria)

- o Serum albumin displaced (causes newborn kernicterus and potentiation of other serum albumin-binders like warfarin)

20. **Anticholinergic side effects** (Know the **ABCD'S** of anticholinergic side effects)

- o **A**norexia
- o **B**lurry vision
- o **C**onstipation/ **C**onfusion
- o **D**ry Mouth
- o **S**edation/ **S**tasis of urine

21. **Aspirin: side effects (ASPIRIN)**
- o **A**sthma
- o **S**alicyalism
- o **P**eptic ulcer disease/ **P**hosphorylation-oxidation uncoupling/ **P**PH/ **P**latelet disaggregation/ **P**remature closure of PDA
- o **I**ntestinal blood loss
- o **R**eye's syndrome
- o **I**diosyncracy
- o **N**oise (tinnitus)

22. **Benzodiazapines: ones not metabolized by the liver (safe to use in liver failure) (LOT)**

- o **L**orazepam
- o **O**xazepam
- o **T**emazepam

23. **Benzodiazepenes: drugs which decrease their metabolism** (I'm Overly Calm)
These drugs increase calming effect of BZDs by reducing metabolism

- o **I**soniazid
- o **O**ral contraceptive pills
- o **C**imetidine

24. Lithium: side effects (LITH)

- **L**eukocytosis
- **I**nsipidus [diabetes insipidus, resulting in polyuria]
- **T**remor/ **T**eratogenesis
- **H**ypothyroidism

25. Organophosphates: effects (If you know these, you will be "LESS DUMB")

- **L**acrimation
- **E**xcitation of nicotinic synapses
- **S**alivation
- **S**weating
- **D**iarrhea
- **U**rination
- **M**icturition
- **B**ronchoconstriction

26. Inhalation anesthetics (SHINE)
- **S**evoflurane
- **H**alothane
- **I**soflurane
- **N**itrous oxide
- **E**nflurane

27. Methyldopa: side effects (METHYLDOPA)
- **M**ental retardation
- **E**lectrolyte imbalance
- **T**olerance
- **H**eadache/ **H**epatotoxicity
- ps**Y**cological upset
- **L**actation in female
- **D**ry mouth
- **O**edema
- **P**arkinsonism
- **A**naemia (haemolytic)

28. Morphine: effects (MORPHINES)

- Miosis
- Orthostatic hypotension
- Respiratory depression
- Pain suppression
- Histamine release/ Hormonal alterations
- Increased ICT
- Nausea
- Euphoria
- Sedation

29. Phenytoin: adverse effects (PHENYTOIN)

- **P**-450 interactions
- **H**irsutism
- **E**nlarged gums
- **N**ystagmus
- **Y**ellow-browning of skin
- **T**eratogenicity
- **O**steomalacia
- **I**nterference with B12 metabolism (hence anemia)
- **N**europathies: vertigo, ataxia, headache

30. Pupils in overdose: morphine vs. amphetamine

(Mor**PHINE**: **Fine**. Am**PHET**amine: **Fat**)
- Mor**phine** overdose: pupils constricted (**fine**).
- Am**phet**amine overdose: pupils dilated (**fat**)

31. Sodium valproate: side effects (VALPROATE)

- **V**omiting
- **A**lopecia
- **L**iver toxicity
- **P**ancreatitis/ **P**ancytopenia
- **R**etention of fats (weight gain)
- **O**edema (peripheral oedema)
- **A**ppetite increase
- **T**remor
- **E**nzyme inducer (liver)

32. SSRIs: side effects (SSRI)

- **S**erotonin syndrome
- **S**timulate CNS
- **R**eproductive dysfunctions in male
- **I**nsomnia

33. Metabolism enzyme inducers (**R**andy's **B**lack **C**ar **G**oes **P**urr **P**urr and **S**mokes)

- **R**ifampin
- **B**arbiturates
- **C**arbamazepine
- **G**risoefulvin
- **P**henytoin
- **P**henobarb
- **S**moking cigarettes

34. Tricyclic antidipressents (TCA): side effects (TCA'S)
- **T**hrombocytopenia
- **C**ardiac (arrhymia, MI, stroke)
- **A**nticholinergic (tachycardia, urinary retention, etc.)
- **S**eizures

35. Antibiotics contraindicated during pregnancy (MCAT)

- **M**etronidazole
- **C**hloramphenicol
- **A**minoglycoside
- **T**etracycline

36. Etoposide: action, indications, side effect (eTOPoside)
- **Action**:
    - Inhibits **TOP**oisomerase II
- **Indications**:
    - **T**esticular carcinoma
    - **O**at cell carcinoma of lung
    - **P**rostate carcinoma

- **Side effect:**
  - Affects **TOP** of your head, causing **alopecia**

37. **Torsades de Pointes: drugs causing (APACHE)**
    - Amiodarone
    - Procainamide
    - Arsenium
    - Cisapride
    - Haloperidol
    - Erythromycin

38. **Respiratory depression inducing drugs (STOP** breathing)

    - Sedatives and hypnotics
    - Trimethoprim
    - Opiates
    - Polymyxins

39. **Teratogenic drugs: major non-antibiotics (TAP CAP)**

    - Thalidomide
    - Androgens
    - Progestins
    - Corticosteroids
    - Aspirin & indomethacin
    - Phenytoin

OBSTETRICS AND GYNECOLOGY

1. **Post-partum haemorrhage (PPH): causes (4 'T's)**

   - Tissue (retained placenta)
   - Tone (uterine atony)
   - Trauma (traumatic delivery, episiotomy)
   - Thrombin (coagulation disorders, DIC)

2. **Preeclampsia: classic triad (PREeclampsia)**

- Proteinuria
- Rising blood pressure
- Edema

3. RLQ pain: brief female differential diagnosis (AEIOU)
- Appendicitis/ Abscess
- Ectopic pregnancy/ Endometriosis
- Inflammatory disease (pelvic)/ IBD
- Ovarian cyst (rupture, torsion)
- Uteric colic/ Urinary stones

4. Ovarian cancer: risk factors ("Blue FILM")

- Breast cancer
- Family history
- Infertility
- Low parity
- Mumps

5. Maternal Alpha-fetoprotein: causes for increased levels during pregnancy (Increased Maternal Serum Alpha Feto Protein)

- Intestinal obstruction
- Multiple gestation/ Miscalculation of gestational age/ Myeloschisis
- Spina bifida cystica
- Anencephaly/ Abdominal wall defect
- Fetal death
- Placental abruption

6. Endometriosis—symptoms (DIPS)
- Deep dyspareunia
- Infertility
- Pelvic pain (cyclical)
- Secondary dysmenorrhea

7. APGAR score components (SHIRT)

- o Skin color: blue or pink
- o Heart rate: below 100 or over 100
- o Irritability (response to stimulation): none, grimace or cry
- o Respirations: irregular or good
- o Tone (muscle): some flexion or active

8. Asherman syndrome features (ASHERMAN)

- o **A**cquired Anomaly
- o **S**econdary to **S**urgery
- o **H**ysterosalpingography confirms diagnosis
- o **E**ndometrial damage/ **E**ugonadotropic
- o **R**epeated uterine trauma
- o **M**issed **M**enses
- o **A**dhesions
- o **N**ormal estrogen and progesterone levels

9. Menopause - symptoms (FSH > 20 IU/L)

One must remember that measurement of the increased FSH levels is the most accurate blood test for the confirmation of menopause.

- o Hot **F**lushes/**F**emale genitalia (vaginal) dryness and burning
- o **S**weats at night
- o **H**eadaches
- o **I**nsomnia
- o **U**rge incontinence
- o **L**ibido decreases

10. CVS and amniocentesis: when performed

- o "Chorionic" has **9** letters and Chorionic villus sampling performed at **9** weeks gestation.
- o "AlphaFetoProtein" has **16** letters and it's measured at **16** weeks gestation.

11. Instrumental delivery prerequisites (AABBCCDDEE)
- o Analgesia
- o Antisepsis
- o Bowel empty

- o **B**ladder empty
- o **C**ephalic presentation
- o **C**onsent
- o **D**ilated cervix
- o **D**isproportion (no CPD)
- o **E**ngaged
- o **E**pisiotomy

12. Gestation period, oocytes, vaginal pH, menstrual cycle: normal numbers

- o 4 is the normal pH of the vagina.
- o 40 weeks is the normal gestation period.
- o 400 oocytes released between menarche and menopause.
- o 400,000 oocytes present at puberty.
- o 28 days in a normal menstrual cycle.
- o 280 days (from last normal menstrual period) in a normal gestation period.

13. Forceps: indications for delivery (FORCEPS)

- o **F**oetus alive
- o **O**s dilated
- o **R**uptured membrane
- o **C**ervix taken up
- o **E**ngagement of head
- o **P**resentation suitable
- o **S**agittal suture in AP diameter of inlet

14. Shoulder dystocia: management (HELPERR)

- o Call for **H**elp
- o **E**pisiotomy
- o **L**egs up [McRoberts position]
- o **P**ressure subrapubically [not on fundus]
- o **E**nter the pelvis maneuvers (internal rotation): such as Rubin II maneuver, Wood's screw maneuver and reverse Wood's screw maneuver
- o **R**emove the posterior arm

- Roll the patient/ Return head into vagina [Zavanelli maneuver] for C-section/ Rupture clavicle or pubic symphysis

15. Smallest Fetal Head Diameter (M T P)

- Bi-Mastoid-7.5
- Bi-Temporal-8.00
- Bi-Parietal-8.5

16. IUGR: causes (IUGR)

- **I**nherited: chromosomal and genetic disorders
- **U**terus: placental insufficiency
- **G**eneral: maternal malnutrition, smoking
- **R**ubella and other congenital infection

17. Multiple pregnancy complications (HI, PAPA)

- **H**ydramnios (Poly)
- **I**UGR
- **P**reterm labour
- **A**ntepartum haemorrhage
- **P**re-eclampsia
- **A**bortion

18. Cardiotocogram (CTG) interpretation (Dr. C. BraVADO)

- **D**efine Risk
- **C**ontractions (in 10 mins)
- **B**aseline Rate (should be 110-160)
- **V**ariability (should be greater than 5)
- **A**ccelerations
- **D**ecelerations
- **O**verall (normal or not)

19. Oral contraceptive complications: warning signs (ACHES)
- **A**bdominal pain
- **C**hest pain

- o Headache (severe)
- o Eye (blurred vision)
- o Sharp leg pain

20. Dystocia: causes (4 Ps)

- o Passenger (large baby)
- o Passage (Abnormal Pelvis)
- o Power (uterine contraction)
- o Proportion (disproportion Cephalo-pelvic)

21. Oral contraceptives: side effects (CONTRACEPTIVES)

- o Cholestatic jaundice
- o Oedema (corneal)
- o Nasal congestion
- o Thyroid dysfunction
- o Raised BP
- o Acne/ Alopecia/ Anaemia
- o Cerebrovascular disease
- o Elevated blood sugar
- o Porphyria/ Pigmentation/ Pancreatitis
- o Thromboembolism
- o Intracranial hypertension
- o Vomiting (progesterone only)
- o Erythema nodosum/ Extrapyramidal effects
- o Sensitivity to light

22. Recurrent miscarriage causes (RIBCAGE)
- o Radiation
- o Immune reaction
- o Bugs (infection)
- o Cervical incompetence
- o Anatomical anomaly (uterine septum etc.)
- o Genetic (aneuploidy, balanced translocation etc.)
- o Endocrine

23. Pelvic Inflammatory Disease: Complications (I FACE PID)

- Infertility
- Fitz-Hugh-Curitis syndrome
- Abscesses
- Chronic pelvic pain
- Ectopic pregnancy
- Peritonitis
- Intestinal obstruction
- Disseminated: sepsis, endocarditis, arthritis, meninigitis

24. Postpartum collapse: causes (HEPARINS)

- Hemorrhage
- Eclampsia
- Pulmonary embolism
- Amniotic fluid embolism
- Regional anaesthetic complications
- Infarction (MI)
- Neurogenic shock
- Septic shock

25. Risk factors for post-partum haemmorrage (PPH): (PARTUM)

- Polyhydroamnios/ Prolonged labour/ Previous cesarean
- APH
- Recent history of bleeding
- Twins
- Uterine fibroids
- Multiparity

26. Secondary amenorrhea: causes (SOAP)
- Stress
- OCP
- Anorexia
- Pregnancy

27. Female pelvis: shapes (GAP)
In order from most to least common:
- Gynecoid

- o **A**ndroid /**A**nthropoid
- o **P**latypelloid

28. Menopause—long-term effects (CONU)

- o **C**ardiovascular disease: IHD, stroke, arterial disease
- o **O**steoporosis: accelerated bone loss leading to osteoporosis and pathological fractures
- o **N**eurological: Alzheimer's disease
- o **U**rogenital atrophy: loss of pelvic floor muscle tone

29. Causes and risk factors of infertility in females (INFERTILE)

- o **I**diopathic
- o **N**o ovulation – PCOS, menopause, pituitary disease, thyroid disorders
- o **F**ibroids – physical hindrance
- o **E**ndometriosis
- o **R**egular bleeding pattern disrupted – oligo/amenorrhoea
- o **T**ubal disease leading to blocked tubes/impaired mobility
- o **I**ncreasing age >35 years
- o **L**arge size – obesity
- o **E**xcessive weight loss – anorexia nervosa

ENDOCRINOLOGY

1. Symptoms of acromegaly (ABCDEF)

- o **A**rthralgia/Arthritis
- o **B**lood pressure raised
- o **C**arpal tunnel syndrome
- o **D**iabetes
- o **E**nlarged organs
- o **F**ield defect

2. Causes of hypernatremia (6 D's)

- o **D**iuretics
- o **D**ehydration
- o **D**iabetes insipidus
- o **D**ocs (iatrogenic)
- o **D**iarrhea
- o **D**isease: kidney, sickle cell, etc.

3. **Symptoms of hypothyroidism (MOM'S SO TIRED)**

- o **M**emory loss
- o **O**besity
- o **M**alar flush/**M**enorrhagia
- o **S**lowness
- o **S**kin and hair become dry
- o **O**nset is gradual
- o **T**ired
- o **I**ntolerance to cold
- o **R**aised blood pressure
- o **E**nergy levels are low
- o **D**epressed

4. **Pheochromocytoma (rule of 10's)**
- o **10%** extra-abdominal
- o **10%** malignant
- o **10%** bilateral
- o **10%** in children
- o **BUT** 30% genetic/syndromic!

5. **Phaeochromocytoma symptoms (4Ps)**

- o **P**ain
- o **P**allor
- o **P**alpitations
- o **P**erspiration

6. **Diabetic ketoacidosis: precipitating factors (5 I's)**

- o **I**nfection

- o Ischaemia (cardiac, mesenteric)
- o Infarction
- o Ignorance (poor control)
- o Intoxication (alcohol)

7. **General principles of diabetic ketoacidosis management (FLIRT)**

- o **FL**uid
- o **I**nsulin drip
- o **R**ule out MI
- o **T**reat underlying cause

8. Adrenal gland: Hormones secreted:

Medulla (MEN)

- o **M**edulla
- o **E**pinephrine
- o **N**orepinephrine

Cortex (Make Good Sweets)

- o **M**ineralocorticoids, (aldosterone)
- o **G**lucocorticoids, (cortisol)
- o **S**ex hormone (androgen)

9. **Symptoms of hyperthyroidism (SWEATING)**

- o **S**weating
- o **W**eight loss
- o **E**motional liability
- o **A**ppetite is increased
- o **T**remor/**T**achycardia due to AF
- o **I**ntolerance to heat/**I**rregular menstruation/**I**rritability
- o **N**ervousness
- o **G**oitre and **G**astrointestinal problems (loose stools/diarrhoea)

10. Insulinoma (rule of 10's)

- **10%** are part of MEN1 syndrome
- **10%** are multiple
- **10%** are malignant
- **10%** contain ectopic pancreatic tissue

11. Causes of Addison's Disease (ADDISON)

- **A**utoimmune (90% cases)
- **D**egenerative (amyloid)
- **D**rugs (ketoconazole)
- **I**nfections (TB, HIV)
- **S**econdary (low ACTH); hypopituitarism
- **O**thers—adrenal bleeding
- **N**eoplasia (secondary carcinoma)

12. Diabetes medication—oral hypoglycaemics (BAGS)

- **B**iguanides
- **A**lpha-glucosidase inhibitors
- **G**litazones (thiazolidinediones)
- **S**ulphonylureas

13. Complications of diabetes mellitus (KEVINS)
- **K**idney: Nephropathy
- **E**ye disease: retinopathy and cataracts
- **V**ascular: coronary artery disease, cerebrovascular disease, peripheral vascular disease
- **I**nfective: TB, recurrent UTIs
- **N**euromuscular; Peripheral neuropathy
- **S**kin: Necrobiosis lipoidica diabeticorum, granuloma annulare, diabetic dermopathy

14. General management of thyroid storm (PCP'S)

MNEMONICS

- **P**TU - 1gm PO
- **C**orticosteroids
- **P**ropranolol
- **S**liding scale insulin

www.ingramcontent.com/pod-product-compliance
Lightning Source LLC
Chambersburg PA
CBHW052236220526
45471CB00001B/61